THE
COLOR OF
EVERYTHING

THE
COLOR of
EVERYTHING

A JOURNEY TO QUIET THE
CHAOS WITHIN

CORY RICHARDS

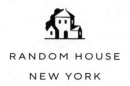

RANDOM HOUSE

NEW YORK

For my family and everything.

For Haliy and everything else.

All ways. Always.

Let everything happen to you

Beauty and terror

Just keep going

No feeling is final

—RAINER MARIA RILKE

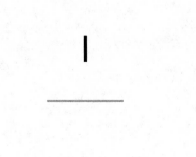

I

1

The past, she is haunted, the future is laced.

—Gregory Alan Isakov

It's December 28, 2010. I wake up in a blue room and panic for a moment because I've forgotten where I am. Curtains with delicate floral patterns and tattered hems bend the shadows of iron bars. The *adhan*, the Muslim call to prayer, moans though the windows. I brush the curtains aside and the damp air and words of the *salāt al-fajr*, the dawn prayer, spill in. Islamabad spreads out below me as clumps of dark shapes, interrupted by dots of orange and green. A streetlight. A kitchen window. A barking dog. The soft, sticky sound of tires on wet pavement. Several blocks away, the minaret of a mosque pierces the sky, illuminated against the darkness, and the muezzin calls out from the too-loud, tinny speakers. I can't understand the words, but I appreciate how they compel a quarter of the world to fall to their knees in prayer five times a day.

Six weeks later, on the side of the thirteenth-highest mountain in the world, I'm praying to anyone who might listen and I remember the *salāt al-fajr*, the first morning in Pakistan, and every morning before it. I'm not religious but this morning I'm being buried alive. I will slowly run out of air and suffocate under the snow. It seems as good a time as any to pray.

They'll find my body in the spring when my orange down suit emerges from the melting snow and feathers float from the tears. After months of uncertainty, Mom and Dad will finally have closure, and all the fights and fuss and anger we endured together will seem silly compared to my death. I wonder if my eyes will be open or closed and if they will still be blue.

These are my thoughts while dying.

Like my childhood, the avalanche becomes sharp fragments of memory as bits of life's strata overlap and blur. A cold blast of snow shoved into my open mouth as I gasp for breath. Snow up my nostrils and down my collar. I'm wet and annoyed that I can't scream because I'm choking. Colorful splinters appear amidst violent flashes of black and white as the weight of my body is sucked deeper into the debris. Down is up. Up is down. Up and down become concepts and concepts are useless in this moment. My joints feel loose and limp in their sockets as fear is replaced by instinct, instinct is replaced by anger, and finally, anger is replaced by resignation. Time dilates and my brain thrashes to make sense of everything. Of anything. One second. One year. A birthday. A date. A bowl of Cheerios. Parking tickets. Song lyrics and books and movies. Faces and things unsaid and words I wish I could unspeak and actions I wish to undo and things I never did, and I remember that I have taxes to pay. I hear Dad say, "Nothing is certain in this world but death and taxes." Life *does* flash before my eyes but there is no poetry to it. It's just Polaroids of a collection of things, emotions, and questions.

My senses expand and blend into a single, encompassing sensation. This is dying. I hear the snow in my mouth and taste blue and smell frozen as everything becomes something different altogether before crashing back into a life unfinished. The fragments get sucked from my brain into a black hole, a singularity. I'm not ready to die. But I *am* dying and no amount of swimming, no god, and no prayer can save me. I summon all the force I have left and thrust my hand and head and life toward what I hope is the sky. *In sha'Allah* . . . if God wills . . .

I stop fifteen seconds and lifetimes later. I'm entirely buried aside from one arm extended and shoved under my chin, cocking my head up toward a gray sky. I'm tangled in purple rope as the snow in my mouth melts and tastes like metal and drips down my throat and I drool. My breath comes in jerking, frenzied gasps that move too quickly to fill my lungs. I free my arm and dig around my head and neck and chest, working frantically to free myself from the snow before another avalanche comes. Simone and Denis are dead and buried and I will leave their bodies under the snow and crawl down the valley alone and I will scream.

I thrash and dig and whimper. Another minute passes before I hear Simone, which doesn't make sense because he's dead and it's too soon for a ghost to be talking to me. Ghosts take time to gestate and find their immaterial voice in the material world. Besides, I don't believe in ghosts—I'm an atheist again. But now the ghost is on top of me and I feel his hands. He's not a panicked hallucination and says, "Cory, everything is okay." I'm alive and everything is okay, yet nothing is okay. I hear another voice step back into the world as Denis says, "Simone! I too am okay!" No one is dead.

I untangle my camera and turn it toward my face as I begin to cry. It's a reflex now. It's all I know how to do to stop my brain when life is going too fast, when it all becomes too big to understand. I am the snow collapsing on itself and I feel myself breaking into a thousand pieces. Maybe a picture can hold them together. The world is small around me as I kneel in the snow on the edge of my own death and cry tears of shock, pain, and relief.

Forty-seven minutes pass. Frozen sweat and tears hang from

my beard in salty globs of ice. My expression is full of confusion and exhaustion and terror. The reflex comes again. I turn the camera on myself and press the shutter five times as I stumble down through the icefall. My legs feel soft. This moment is a single grain of sand and will be suspended forever in the neck of the hourglass of my life. I am at once the same and different as overlapping versions of myself—my life bisected by a great swath of snow.

For those of you who are here for adventure and climbing and pictures, that's all in here, but this is not a book about that. It is a story of me, and a story about the stories we tell ourselves. It's about the brain and the heart: mine and maybe yours. It's a story of the binaries that draw us to the middle. It is black and white and right and wrong and joy and despair. It is success and failure and madness. It is the before and the after and everything in between.

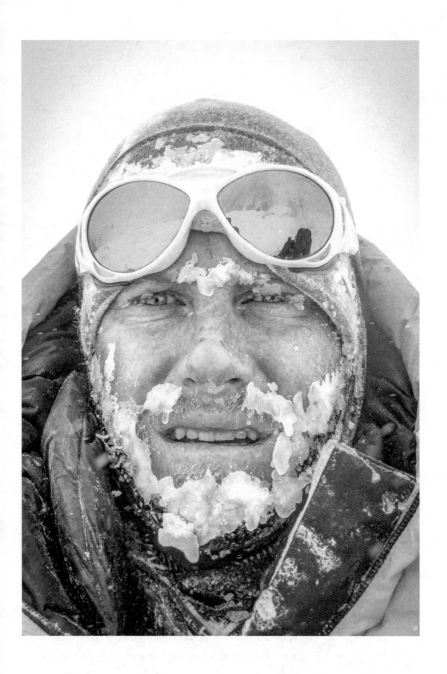

2

Let the wild rumpus start!

—Maurice Sendak, *Where the Wild Things Are*

My birth is miraculous in the way that they all are. The probability that I exist is 1 in $10^{2,685,000}$, which is to say a lot had to happen before late May 1981. The way I understand it, there was a big explosion that sent atoms careening through time and space like celestial buckshot, cascading over each other and coming together as stars and gases and planets and moons and asteroids. And then lightning struck, or God called out, or a great sea turtle crawled from the ocean, and life happened. Billions of years and at least as many unlikely coincidences later, I crawled into the world.

From the beginning of time until now, with all the innumerable events that happened just so, I am very improbable. Just 1 in $10^{2,685,000}$. I know this because Dad teaches math. He'll also tell me that the improbability of my existence doesn't make me any more special than anyone else. In fact, it makes us equal because we all share an identical unlikelihood. And still, I choose to believe that a spring day is miraculous because the alternative is to believe it isn't and that just seems boring considering the prodigious amount of everything that came together as me. But this isn't a math book. It's the story of my life, which started the way all others do: screaming and crying and covered in blood.

Mom tells the story of my birth in broad, impressionistic strokes and I fill in the blanks with vivid details that are probably all wrong. I see it like a movie, with many large people looming over my head and Dad is somehow Hugh Grant. There is confusion and tiny beads of sweat across a peaked young brow and pursed lips spitting air in short, rhythmic bursts. There's chaos and a wheelchair with a wheel that rattles back and forth as it tries to keep up with the others. Mom screams at Dad, "I'll never forgive you for this!" while he brushes hair from her forehead and knows that the best way to support her is to say nothing at all.

One person wants my skin to be clean. One person holds me by my feet and breaks the tether to my mom with a surgical clamp. Someone inexplicably wants to steal the foreskin of my penis (a transgression for which I harbor some anger). Another moves me onto Mom's chest, and everyone is saying "welcome" and "shhhh" but I don't want to shush. I never have and I never will.

A red second hand ticks and says 3:41 A.M. A doctor in blue asks, "Is he breathing?," which is a stupid question. Why would they be telling me "shhhh" if I wasn't? I imagine already being annoyed with adults as a warm, rubbery hand on the back of my neck cradles my wet, purple skin. Strands of blond hair are pasted against my scalp with afterbirth, and I stare at the blue hospital gowns and yellow lights and red second hand, unable to define them because I can't yet see color. There are many sounds, and everything is too bright and I feel like I'm not fully baked, as if my skin is too thin and sensitive. I'll always feel this way. I try to get used to the feeling of using my lungs, gasping to make sense of everything. But I never will. This is the only thing I'm sure is true from the story of my birth.

Mom is called Kit—her college friends are allowed to call her
Kitty, but no one else. She has sandy blond hair and sharp features that make her strong and elegant. When she thinks, and
she's always thinking, she twists a wayward strand and brushes it
between her lips and stares. Her eyes are hazel and they like to
read. She's 5'4" and slight with light olive skin and freckles on
her arms. Her fingers are thin and bony. She drinks hot water.
She loves bourbon and salted caramel ice cream and gives me her
nose, her jaw, cheekbones, and wrists. She calls me "honey" and
"sweetheart" and "Cor" and says things like "Oh dear . . ." and "It
is what it is."

Dad hates his first name and goes by his middle name and
introduces himself as "Court, as in traffic" because he's funny and
loves words. He has light brown hair and a small red mole on his
right cheek. His face is round and shaved shiny for the winters
when he isn't allowed to have facial hair because his weekend job
as a ski patroller forbids it. During the summers when he works
construction and wears a worn leather tool belt, a white T-shirt,
and jeans, he lets his beard grow and the hair is blond and full
and slightly wavy and he looks like a Greek Stoic named Epicu-
rus. He doesn't know it, but he's an Epicurean disciple and navi-
gates the world in ataraxia, a Stoic word for a state free from
distress or worry. He has a hairy chest where I sleep as a baby and
paw at the soft strands and drool and reach up and put my fingers in his mouth. He loves beer and *gelato al limone.* He gives me
his blue eyes, his skin, his ears, his legs, and his feet with awkwardly bent long toes that curve outward. He calls me "Cor Por"
and loves to sing and whistle classical music. He says things like
"This too shall pass." He rarely says "I love you." And more than
any other phrase, he says "Go gently," reminding us that the
world is best navigated with grace.

Mom is polite and well mannered because she comes from Minnesota, where they value tablecloths and porcelain. Her family photographs look like outtakes from *Bewitched*, where everything has a place and men wear suits and women wear pearls. Her dad was a World War II veteran who flew PBY planes over the Pacific and rescued other men whose planes crashed in the aqua-blue water. But he never talked about it because that wasn't what men of his generation did. Her mother kept a tidy home, and they belonged to a country club where the family played tennis and golf and wore white.

On family vacations, Mom and her four siblings skied at Buck Hill and visited a small cabin that smelled of cedar and mildew in the dark, mossy woods that surround Lake Superior. They drove across the county in a heavy station wagon to the Tetons and climbed Baxter's Pinnacle and exchanged tennis rackets for leather hiking boots. Through the windows, they watched shaggy bison meander through fields of sage while listening to my grandpa talk about the importance of wild places. And she knew that while her body belonged to the Lake Country, her heart belonged to the West.

When she was in college at Wellesley, she studied art history and philosophy and spent two summers at Lake O'Hara Lodge in the Canadian Rockies, exchanging the pressed linens of her childhood for wool knickers and hemp ropes while she learned to climb mountains and glaciers. When she graduated, she moved west to Utah, following State Highway 210 to its end at a township called Alta.

Dad grew up on the east bench of the Salt Lake Valley in a single-story home with sharp granular sand in the stucco walls.

From the porch, he could see the light array on top of the Walker Bank Building illuminating the night sky with the weather forecast: solid blue for clear skies, flashing blue for clouds, red for rain, and flashing red for snow.

Downtown Salt Lake City was mostly asphalt, but the roads where Dad lived were still dirt and he watched the paving trucks lumber through the dust, sealing the earth with long black seams. When he was six, he watched five finches get trapped in the tar, becoming more and more stuck as they flapped for freedom. The road workers eventually cleaved off their heads with the dull edges of their shovels, teaching Dad an overlapping lesson of violence and mercy.

As the pavement expanded, his innocence was slowly buried under asphalt, swallowed as all childhoods eventually are. But the earth protested, bending and warping the pavement with roots and blades of grass that pushed up through the cracks, and he learned that wildness was not something that can ever be tamed.

In the 1950s, Salt Lake City was the helm of Mormon culture, and the Richards family was, by all accounts, Mormon royalty. Dad's great-great-grandfather Willard Richards was instrumental in the development of the church. He was present at the lynching and murder of Mormonism's founding prophet, Joseph Smith, hiding behind a door and escaping through a window. Dad smiles and we come from a long line of cowards.

But he didn't have much time for the Mormon God and left the church at sixteen in search of a new faith. He found it in 1959 when he read *Starlight and Storm* by the French mountaineer Gaston Rébuffat. He saw himself mirrored in stories of counterculture climbers who wore thick beards and smoked hand-rolled cigarettes and climbed the big mountain faces of the Alps. The ashlar granite of the Mormon Temple was replaced by cathedrals of uncut stone and ice. Guidebooks and mountain literature became his scriptures because climbing was his new religion. In search of mountains, he too followed State Highway 210 to its end and the place where the story of our family begins.

Founded as an outpost to house silver miners in 1865, Alta, Utah, boomed until the ore was exhausted and an avalanche destroyed the skeletal remains of the bunkhouses and saloons, leaving a sole resident as the keeper of the town. In order to escape back taxes on mining claims, George Watson donated the land he owned to the U.S. Forest Service with the caveat they use it to build a ski area. Alta opened its first ski lift in 1938.

When Mom and Dad met in 1970, Alta was a mix of hippies, tourists, hermits, and a handful of old-timers who might as well have been miners with unnaturally long life because Alta is timeless. It has gravity and pride and it's hard to tell if people there are lost or trapped or free. Mom made beds at the dimly lit Rustler Lodge, which smelled like wet socks and the dry smoke from the fireplaces that cast orange rectangles on the pillows of snow outside. Dad worked on the ski patrol and smelled like Winston Filters, ski boots, and gunpowder from the bombs he threw to set off avalanches.

They fell in love when he found her in a midmountain restaurant with frozen toes and he removed her ski boots, placing her feet against his hairy chest. To Mom, this is *the* moment, the brink over which she poured headlong into love. They were twenty-two and twenty-six and hopeful.

Because men were forbidden in the girls' dorms, Dad usually escaped her room through the window into the early morning, walking back to his bunkhouse guarded against the cold by the warm afterglow of love and a cigarette. They perfected this dance over two years, weaving themselves together over days and nights that eventually became the seamless duality of love.

On June 3, 1972, Mom and Dad exchanged vows on the short

green grass behind my grandparents' house on North Ferndale Road in Wayzata, Minnesota. A string quartet played late into the night accompanied by crickets.

They spent the early years of marriage in a disjointed traverse of the American West. Dad followed Mom over countless miles of ski slopes and trails and listened more than he talked. He watched her dissect the world as they huddled under granite boulders to escape the rain and lightning. They made friends. They got drunk on Jack Daniel's in flooded tents and ate cheese and salami and made love. They screamed at each other and cried. He cleaned his nails with the small blade of a Swiss Army pocketknife and built tiny piles of dirt before blowing them away while Mom peered over the top of a book and held her tongue. They noticed the undulations of geology in landscapes and guessed the distance of straight stretches of road as if the West was unfolding just for them. And after six years of wandering and discovery, the aggregate of their love swelled in her belly.

My brother was born in the spring of 1979 after a painful, days-long labor. His eyes eventually settled to a hazel that I often remember as molasses. He wears Mom's light olive skin but otherwise looks like Dad and arrived in the world mercurial, ready, and self-assured. He is mysterious with dark brown hair and round features. I will love him, but our relationship will always be complicated.

After he was born, Mom was struck with a sticky sadness. She loved him completely but was blocked by moderate postpartum depression (PPD) that contracted her ability to emotionally connect. She barely slept and went straight back to work to anchor herself, compounding the already overwhelming stress of being a new parent.

PPD is commonly a multigenerational experience that cascades from mother to child, over and over. It's one of many fibers spun down through generations. After all, family dynamics aren't independent clusters of choice and consequence, but rather a tapestry of intricately woven threads of action and reaction, passing over and under each other, knotting together time, emotion, and experience as one.

One of the most common results of PPD is insecure attachments, a pattern of connection that mirrors the insecurity felt in the emotional bond between caregiver and child. People with insecure attachments can be clingy and can ignore and otherwise confuse interactions with everyone based on the fear of abandonment or rejection . . . because that's what the emotional disconnect of PPD teaches is inevitable.

Mom fought the depression with work, distracting herself from emotional turmoil while reinforcing her autonomy. Because of their schedules, Dad assumed the role of daily caregiver for my brother during his most fragile months, carrying him in a chest harness and on the back of his bike while forging an unbreakable bond. Neither of my parents believed that motherhood was a one-dimensional existence. But Utah told them something different: that working made her a bad mother. So, under her breath, she said, "Screw 'em" and somehow made it elegant while Dad changed diapers.

By the time I'm born two years later, Mom is the breadwinner in a house of boys. Because PPD is sticky, she dips a bit again after my birth, struggling to balance two young boys and the living that keeps us alive. We don't have money. But we're never hungry and never cold.

I don't remember the first time I go to a therapist because I'm one year old when Mom brings me into the office and says, "I don't know what's wrong. He just seems . . . sad." She's confusing statements with questions, asking if something is broken. I'm a hard baby and they say "colicky," "fussy," and "temperamental" and switch me to soy formula wondering if it's the milk. But nothing really changes. The therapist sits across from us and tells her not to worry and that nothing's broken. Mom looks down at me and worries all the same while I look up at her and cry and she says, "Shhhh." Somehow, she knows. But no one knows exactly what that is.

I drink from the water hose on hot days and live in a colorful montage of memories with no connective tissue. I eat dog food. I shit my pants. I learn how to ride a bike and crash it and bleed from my skull. Ice cream trucks. Hot white pavement at an aquablue swimming pool. Grilled cheese with Kraft singles. The back seat of the blue Suburban. Dog hair and the smell of a golden retriever. Wrestling with my brother. Fists, fat lips, tears, and time-out. Fresh cherries from the tree. Cherries rotting underfoot.

Sometimes I look at my small feet with bent toes and am washed over by déjà vu as if I've watched these cherries rot before, standing under the same tree in a different time. It comes in waves and hits me as I stare down at my grandmother's meatloaf or as I tiptoe across a hot surface. It's especially strong in moments of boredom and heat, when time slows and I'm unburdened by preoccupation and left with myself. But along with the déjà vu there is a second feeling that I have no way to describe and it will stay with me forever.

A long time from now, I'll learn the word *hiraeth*, which describes a longing and homesickness for a place that can't be returned to. It's the missing of something irretrievably lost or that never existed at all. Maybe all children feel this the moment we leave the womb and come crashing into the world. And maybe these quiet moments are what Mom sees that no one else can. But it's undeniable. There's something different. I'm mercurial and polar and have a sense of being on the outside looking in. I'm as quiet as I am loud, as sweet as I am difficult, and Mom and Dad never really know which version of me will sit down to eat. But I'm too little to give it words.

We live in a two-story, pink-brick Victorian house on Second Avenue with a painted tile that says "Kit e Court" and I think my parents' names sound good together. In the summer, thick ivy grows up the walls and makes the house look magical and full, but Dad says the ivy eats the bricks. He says it's a "pain in the ass." In the fall and winter, when it browns and falls away, the house looks naked and dead, as if it's haunted. I'd rather have a beautiful pain in the ass than a naked and haunted house of ease. I think beautiful things make life better because even if they cause problems, you can always just sit down and look at them, and then maybe the problems won't seem so big after all.

The house is almost a hundred years old, which I take great pride in telling everyone because a hundred years is a long time when you've only been alive for six. The Salt Lake summers are hot and long and I don't like the way the grass in the front yard browns and gets crunchy because it hurts my bare feet. The lawn in the back never seems to brown, though, hidden behind an old brick wall and a large wooden gate that squeaks on its hinges. There's a peach tree with spindly arms that hang over a dog-house. There's a large garage full of things like table saws and nails and hammers and coffee cans full of miscellaneous parts that Dad uses to fix things. He likes to tinker to avoid the clatter of two boys.

Next to the garage is the evergreen backyard, a sandbox, a deck, and a cherry tree that is particularly good for climbing. Behind the garage is a patch of grass where the dog does her business and Dad goes out with a shovel and scrapes the shit from the grass, which seems to make more of a mess than it cleans. Here, the green grass does get brown.

Mom makes chicken breasts and steamed broccoli that she likes to dip in mayonnaise and we eat at a modest table in the kitchen. After dinner, while Dad does the dishes, she sits at a mahogany table in the dining room, which my brother and I aren't allowed in so we don't add crayon art to the walls. This is the room the grown-ups use for dinner parties. She moves the candles to make room for neatly stacked folders she's brought home from her office, where she raises money for the University of Utah. The Development Office phone number is 581-3723 and I call every afternoon to tell her that everything is okay and my brother and I are not dead.

The folders spread out in front of her lean fingers as she makes lists in elegant cursive on personalized notepads that say "From the Office of Kit Richards." The words on the pads are printed in her favorite shade of crimson. She prefers black ballpoint pens that leave a stream of thick ink that smears if you touch it too soon, to which she says, "Shit . . ." and then says "Oops" and covers her mouth. Mom and Dad tell us not to swear but we learn to speak like sailors anyway. It's our own little language of rebellion and a way to say "fuck you" to the overly sanitized way that the Mormons talk. I wonder if Mom and Dad secretly love our foul little mouths.

My brother reads while I draw a disproportional horse-giraffe with extreme birth defects and a swayback so deep that the body looks like a U. I draw scenes from the American West with strange creatures, poorly proportioned cowboys with mashed faces, and oblong Indians, entranced by the feathers, beads, and headdresses of a world of ritual and mystery.

"Wow!" Mom says as she looks at the best goat-cow-giraffe-zebra-horse that's ever been drawn, and we all know I'm destined for greatness. She hangs it on the fridge next to Christmas cards and a shopping list. "Wow!" she says again. "Just wow!"

Now I'm skeptical because even I know it's not that good. My pride crumbles and I start crying sloppy tears. "Honey! What's wrong?" Mom says, and looks at Dad with big eyes and mouths, "What the fuck?" He shrugs and mouths back, "I don't know." This is normal. I cry at a mouse fart. I hyperventilate and suck my bottom lip into my mouth with deep breaths and stutter, "The back is too bent and the neck, the neck, is too long and you hate it!" and she can't help but laugh. But her laughter makes it worse and I scream, *"You hate it!"* She stops laughing because I've gone from sweet to ballistic on a hair trigger. I stomp back to my art supplies and start drawing so hard it tears through the paper and scratches the wood underneath. Unsatisfied with my reaction, I stab the table in frustration and leave a hole that I'll always see. I thunder away when Mom sends me to my room. My brother sits quietly, invisible.

Every Friday in summer, Mom comes home from work and packs duffels and canvas tote bags, puts her three boys in the car, and we drive 100 miles into the Uinta Mountains. When we arrive two hours later, my brother and I are asleep, pulled from the truck in gangly heaps and laid down in bunk beds. Our cabin on the bank of the east fork of the Bear River is an insecure chalet of overconfident kindling hugging itself around a central stone fireplace. On windy nights, I lie awake and listen to the porous walls whistle and moan.

The air here is always colder and smells like pine trees and dirt. Tiny wild strawberries grow around the fire pit just outside the screen door that slams too loud. Dad usually has a chain saw or axe in his hand and always seems to be covered in sawdust with grease on his hands and a sweat mark around his belly button. He builds a deck, bed frames, and a fire-heated hot tub that looks like a witch's cauldron. At night, I watch Mom and Dad slip out of their clothes and into the steaming water, leaning their heads back and saying "Ahhhhhhhh."

When we wake up on Saturday, my brother and I put on fatigues and pretend military equipment and bushwhack endlessly through meadows and willows. With plywood M-16s firmly in grip, we patrol the killing fields of an imaginary war. We ford the river and lie in the wet grass, spying on unsuspecting people in the campground and mimic hand signals that we've seen in movies. My brother tells me to flank the enemy on the right until we're both in position. On his count, we spring from the trees and make machine gun fire noises and scare the shit out of campers who are just trying to enjoy their coffee. They are the first casualties of our war games.

A blue tendril of smoke rising from the chimney guides us home at dusk, covered in mud and mosquito bites, victorious and bruised. We shower and put on Dad's old T-shirts, which hang to our elbows and knees, and Mom says, "Brush your teeth!"

I flip the little hourglass and watch the sand begin to build a tiny mountain while I make an exaggerated grin and foam drips down my chin and onto Dad's shirt.

Dad opens the door to our bunk room at 5:30 A.M. and trumpets his own lyrics to reveille: "Oh lazy Cory, it's time to get up, it's time to get up in the morning!" We gather our skiing equipment and pile into the car and park thirty minutes later just below Bald Mountain Pass where the road is hedged by walls of snow left in the wake of enormous winter avalanches.

We pull on our skiing clothes and boots and strap our skis to tiny packs while listening to Metallica's . . . *And Justice for All,* which Mom has no idea how we got our hands on. She worries the music will make us worship Satan, but not enough to take it away. In any case, she's not with us and Dad doesn't believe in Satan. If anything, the prolific sawing of electric guitars seems to propel us up the 1,500-foot ascent.

We start climbing just as the sun hits the summit of Bald Mountain, inching its way down as we scrape up. Dad teaches us to walk in crampons, the spikes we fix to the bottom of our boots. He puts ice axes in our hands and shows us how to stop ourselves in case we fall. We exhale clouds of hot breath surrounded by black pine trees and walk in silence. Eventually we cross from the cool shadows into the yellow light and the trees become green. Soon we're drenched in sweat and Dad teaches us that sweating can be deadly because it can lead to dehydration and hypothermia. Every day is a school day in the mountains.

The climb is long and my brother is always hundreds of feet ahead, charging upward while I'm lost in my own daydreams of grandeur, imagining the mountain to be a massive Himalayan peak like the pictures from the books that line our staircase at home.

Dad watches us from below and my brother becomes my guide, dropping his voice to a more manly pitch and calling back to make sure I'm okay or instructing me where there is ice or a dangerous step. He stomps out a platform just below the upper cliffs that guard the summit and waits for me while he puts on his skis. But once I arrive and our boots are locked in, he's gone, skidding and carving over the melting snow. I love the ascent. He loves the descent. We are two sides of the same coin. As our muscles and identities and egos grow, fueled by burgeoning hormones, sibling rivalry, and a simmering adolescent rage in both of us, the sweetness of these days will dissolve. But for now, we ski down, put our gear in the back of the car, and drive back to the cabin headbanging to Metallica, untouched by Satan.

On Sundays at the cabin, after all the snow has melted and summer is starting to feel long, we wake up and Mom makes scrambled eggs. Dad burns toast so black that it smokes and says, "Ouch . . . dammit . . ." The smoke alarm goes off as he licks his fingers as Mom waves a dirty dish towel overhead.

"Jesus, Court. Does it have to be on fire to be done?"

"Yes."

We drive twenty-five minutes to a Boy Scout camp on a lake with a blocky quartzite crag that rises above a boulder field. Dad pulls ropes and slings and metal bits from his backpack and ties harnesses around our waists. Mom lies out on a rock and reads Dick Francis novels while Dad walks around the backside of the cliff and throws a rope over the edge, securing it at the top to a tree. For the next eight hours all we do is climb and learn to move over stone.

He teaches us how to trust tiny edges that seem too small to hold any weight. He shows us how to place pieces of metal in the rock to protect us from hitting the ground if we fall. He bends and twists and snakes the rope through itself and makes us memorize a dozen knots until we can do them with our eyes closed. We repeat the routine until one day he doesn't take the rope to the top of the cliff, reminding us that serious climbs don't magically have a safety cord hanging from the summit. Instead, we must learn to climb from the bottom up, dragging the ropes behind. In climbing, this is called "leading."

Dad uses a construction pencil to draw a shitty picture on a paper bag with grease spots and explains the numbers and math. "If you are two feet above the last piece of protection you put in the crack and you fall, you'll go a total of four feet. If you're five feet above the last piece, you'll fall ten feet. Make sense?" In theory, I think. But I'm also about to learn that theory is all well and good, but reality is an asshole.

It all seems perfectly sane at first. My brother belays me, feeding rope out through a device on his harness that will catch me if I fall. I place one piece of protection in a crack and Dad eyes it. He nods approvingly but asks, "Is it good?"

"I think so . . ."

"Better to know so." So I check it again and my forearms begin to ache because I'm holding on too tight. I climb a few more feet and put another piece of protection in another crack and Dad asks, "Is it good?" I grunt and he grunts and smiles and I climb higher, putting in more and more pieces until the lousy 15 feet between me and the ground looks like at least 1,000.

"Jump off."

"What?" my brother and I say at the same time.

Mom says, "Court . . ."

Dad says, "It's fine. Just let go," and my legs start to shake.

"But what if the protection doesn't hold?"

"You said it looked good. Trust it."

"But what if he drops me?" I look at my brother over my shoulder and then back at Dad.

"He won't."

Mom's sitting up now and saying, "Courtney! Don't make him do it if he isn't ready. Cory, it's okay." Despite her concern, Dad is verging on glee. "Don't give him any more rope until he jumps off." This instruction gives my brother great joy and I can tell he's smiling as he gently begins to increase tension on the cord, slowly pulling me off the wall. Now, very calmly, Dad says, "Cory. You're holding on too tight." He too knows more than he knows he knows.

Both my legs are shaking. My hands are sweating and my forearms are screaming and my brother is smiling and Dad is annoyingly calm and Mom is clenching as my fingers that look just like hers start to slide off the rock and I know that this will be the end of everything.

I will fall and there will be blood and Mom will be crying and

Dad will cradle me in his arms and tell me, "Shhhh" and "Don't go," while my brother rocks in the fetal position. I'll leave the world as I entered: screaming, crying, and covered in blood. There will be a funeral where they'll speak of my unimaginable bravery in the face of death—"He was such a courageous boy . . ."—and Metallica will play and they'll name this cliff after me. But the tragedy of my loss will drive an emotional wedge between my parents and Mom won't be able to forgive Dad and she'll leave. Eventually Mom will remarry and my brother will spend alternating weeks between homes and Dad will begin to drink while his beard grows out of control. He'll start smoking again as his walls fill up with shitty drawings on paper bags with long equations that all end in question marks: "How did I miscalculate?" He'll dive into despair until the courts deem him unfit to parent and my poor brother will be removed from the house and become a crack addict, traumatized by a broken home. All the Mormons will say, "It's that devil music and poor parenting. You know the father left the church as a teenager and the poor mother had to work a full-time job. . . ."

The future is written as I feel my fingers finally slip off. There is only the cold hard reality of my tragic end and the last words I'll ever hear are "Jesus, Court!" and I imagine Mom crossing herself as I fly through the air.

But Dad is good at math and no more than four feet later the rope catches me and I hang on my perfect knot while my brother laughs. I keep waiting to hit the ground because the tragedy in my brain was so much more glamorous than the fall I took. There is no blood or ambulance and Mom and Dad remain married and my brother doesn't turn to street drugs to overcome his immeasurable sadness. Dad keeps shaving and doesn't start smoking again, because my brain is very good at creating catastrophes that don't exist.

My brother lowers me to the ground as I wipe tears from my face and dry-heave from the adrenaline of the tiniest climbing fall ever taken. Dad unties the rope and says, "Good job." My brother lowers his voice and says stoically, "My turn," and climbs and falls without tears or fear and I wonder if anyone got divorced or became a drug addict in his head.

I can still feel the salt on my cheeks as we walk back to the car. My brother gleefully swings a dead stick against a tree and it explodes while Mom and Dad hold hands and she laughs about something just for them. I watch them hold tightly to the waning moments of this enchanted childhood. It is a sweet, magical world.

Dad points the car toward Salt Lake and I fall asleep in the back seat and dream of my bravery and 1,000-foot fall, wondering if they'll name the cliff after me anyway. We park in the driveway at home and I notice the green ivy on the house has started to brown. The glory of summer has burned too hot, and fall is coming. Mom says, "Oh dear . . . ," and Dad says, "This too shall pass."

3

Children are not things to be molded,

but are people to be unfolded.

—Jess Lair

In the elevator, Mom checks her watch and pushes 6. The button lights up orange behind chipped paint as soft jazz wafts around us. We ride in silence while I kick the bottom of my skateboard and let it bounce back against my toes until the elevator dings. The waiting room is new but the same as every other with water-damaged *Newsweek* and *National Geographic* magazines on the table. The lady with short hair behind the counter says, "He'll be with you shortly. Just take a seat."

Mom sits next to me in Dr. Doug Goldsmith's office and explains that she's concerned about my behavior. I scan the room and stare at a big book with the letters *DSM III* on the spine and try to pronounce it as a word. Dissum. Dee-esum? The letters are an acronym for *The Diagnostic and Statistical Manual of Mental Disorders*. But for psychologists and therapists, *DSM* translates to "the holy bible" and is the manual for all the ways the brain blows gaskets and goes sideways.

The purple hue cast by tinted windows makes the city look hazy and hot. I sit in silence and pick at my baggy pants. I'm ten years old and destined to be an international superstar skateboarder like Tony Hawk and my bright pink board proves that I'm serious and bound for greatness. My oversized sweatshirt has a large skull on it and Mom is worried that Metallica is finally taking its toll, even though I much prefer Guns N' Roses now. Doug doesn't say much while Mom explains that I'm fighting every authority figure in my life. *"No! I'm not!"* I interrupt. She purses her lips and gives Doug a pointed look. He asks if she can give a specific example of my defiance. "Well, I mean, it's just everything!"

"*See!* You can't even tell him what I'm doing wrong!" I interrupt again. Mom looks at Doug. She doesn't have to say anything because I'm proving her point for her. I don't know why, but all I want to do is fight, which is fostering a near-constant battle between my parents and brother and me. Wash the dishes. No. Bedtime. No. Brush your teeth. No.

In our house, ten years old isn't beyond the reach of a bare-assed walloping and Dad has enormous hands that land with an incredible clap. As much as I want to think the skulls on my clothes make me tough, I still scream in a crystal-shattering pitch when I'm getting spanked. But for me that's almost the point. I want the pain to be heard. If there's a spanking taking place, I want the neighbors to mistake it for murder and call the cops and say, "Oh, that poor boy. Have you seen his father's hands?"

Even the smallest conflicts have a way of turning into major events and Mom tells Doug about a recent argument over dinner, though neither of us can remember what it was about. When I pushed my plate aside and refused to eat, Mom and Dad reminded me that I live in *their* home and certain rules are inflexible. My response was simple: "So it's not my home too? I'm not part of the family? You hate me? Well, I hate you and I'll just fucking leave!"

"Okay, leave." Dad was calling my bluff.

"Fuck your carrots!"

I ran to my room and shoved my survival provisions in my pack, stomped downstairs, and slammed the front door. After putting three blocks between me and the house I started to wonder where I was going and realized that running away requires a plan. It's very easy to be certain amidst comfort. It's easy to fight when consequences are still just abstractions. Seeing that I had nowhere to go, I sat in the neighborhood cemetery and felt the moisture from the wet, manicured lawn soak through my pants. I stretched my hoodie over my knees and rested my chin on the fabric and bounced my head. The headstones spread out as pale blue tiles reflecting the moonlight and I wondered how long it would take for my parents to weep to the news cameras about their lost boy whom they treated so poorly, begging for help to bring him home.

"If you have any information or have seen this boy, please contact the local authorities," the reporter would say. But I would be on a merchant vessel sailing the Atlantic, nameless and muscular. I'd be living in a cabin in the forest, chopping wood without a shirt on. I'd be living in the French Alps in a chalet, painting tortured canvases and making love to foreign women like the ones I saw in Playboy. *Years would pass and I'd be a bear of a man before I returned home, chiseled from stone. I'd have a beard and long hair and tattoos. Mom would finally exhale after decades and weep at my feet and apologize while Dad would put his hand on the back of my neck and say, "Welcome home, son . . . we never should've made you eat your vegetables."*

I sat in the cemetery for an hour before realizing that I didn't have a sleeping bag or anything else that I might really need but instead had filled my bag with a sketchbook and clothes and fruit snacks. Defeated but still defiant, I walked back home. Mom was sitting on the couch and Dad was correcting papers. There were no news cameras to be seen.

"How was it?" Dad asked as Mom sat silently.

"I forgot my sleeping bag. I just came back to grab it."

"That'll get ya. It's in the garage." I considered grabbing it and hitchhiking to Alaska. But it was warm inside and the fruit snacks were already gone. Instead, I walked upstairs and went to bed without brushing my teeth. I could run away tomorrow.

When I woke up, my backpack was still packed, ready to cast off at a moment's notice. I smelled breakfast and wandered downstairs, where my brother was eating apple cinnamon oatmeal and burnt toast. The microwave dinged and Dad brought me the plate of vegetables I refused to eat the night before and cheerfully said, "Here's your breakfast, Cor Por! Oh, I grabbed your sleeping bag from the garage for you. It's just by the door."

Back in Doug's office, it all seems so stupid now as Mom calmly explains that this was just one example of many. "We could tell him that the sky is blue and he'll reject it. He'll question the nature of what blue *means*. How the hell are we supposed to get him to eat his peas when he's answering with existentialism? And then he just runs away . . ." She lets her hands fall in her lap while her shoulders hunch forward and I wonder what existentialism is.

Recently the feeling of being on the outside looking in has intensified to the point of invisibility. I feel like I'm yelling through glass but no one looks up. That my life can look so perfect from the exterior and feel so chaotic within seeds a deep sense of guilt, as though by living at all, I'm doing something wrong. Or at least I just can't get it right.

At first I only rejected my immediate family. But soon I began to offer my defiance to everyone. Now no one holds enough authority to escape my rebellion. I've decided that to protest and defy is to be seen, and to be seen is to be loved.

Doug asks Mom if she might sit outside for a few minutes.

She touches me on the back of the head and I hear delicate bracelets fall around her wrist. The door closes and I start crying.

Doug hands me a box of tissues and I brace for him to tell me all the things I'm doing wrong. Instead, he says nothing for a long time, waiting for me to cry out the reservoir or use up the tissues . . . whichever comes last.

"Your brother is a pretty good skateboarder, I bet."

"Yeah."

"Do you want to be like him?"

"Yeah."

It's such a simple line of questioning that I'm annoyed. I can't see that he's pulling a thread in a tapestry that predates me and one that's so subtle it will be twenty-eight years before it all starts to make sense. It goes something like this:

Sleep deprivation, stress, career, and motherhood are all a bit overwhelming and despite all of the love in the world, there is a disconnect between my mom and brother. It's no one's fault. It's so subtle that no one can see it at all. And then, almost exactly two years later, my brother is told, "Meet your little brother. What was once all yours is now shared. Play nice." In an instant three lives became four and those four lives intertwined to create a fifth entity: the Richards.

As I'm writing this chapter, I call Dad to figure out how many relationships are possible in a family of four and he tells me the equation is $N \times (N-1) / 2 = R$, where N is the number of family members and R is the number of relationships. I ask him to do the math because I'm allergic to algebra, and he says the answer is six. But because I live through my eyes, I make a list instead so I can *see* the relationships and it looks like this:

1. Mom & Dad
2. Mom & me

3. Dad & me
4. My brother & me
5. Mom & brother
6. Dad & brother
7. Mom & Dad & me
8. Mom & my brother & me
9. Dad & my brother & me
10. Mom & dad & my brother
11. Us

Mathematically, Dad says this doesn't make sense and I tell him that's because his numbers only account for the relationship between two individuals, but that isn't how families work. Family dynamics are confusing, and each baby complicates them exponentially. He says that there are only six possible relationships and I ask him to tell me which of the relationships I've listed don't exist. He can't and says, "What are we missing?"

Twenty-eight years ago, Doug is calculating relationships too, trying to understand a cast of characters and levers of emotion that are disrupting what should be a blissful childhood. Doug is panning for psychological gold and I'm thinking about the big book on the shelf and wondering what it says about brothers who are too close to separate.

Mom and Dad put skis on our feet and ropes in our hands, taught us to shoot bows and arrows, and enrolled us in team sports. We strap firecrackers to toy soldiers, throw rotten peaches at each other, and race up the same cherry tree, vying to be the one who touches the top first. My brother sits on my shoulders and slaps me in the face with my own hands and says, "Why are you hitting yourself? Why are you hitting yourself?" He lets long strings of spit drip from his mouth until they hang inches above my face. I scream and he sucks it all back up.

We've done all the same things, but as we're growing up, there is only room for one champion. Sibling rivalry is normal and we are normal until one day we aren't. We're both drinking from the same emotional well, too close and too entwined, so neither of us feels like we can stand out. Anger grows. He still sits on my shoulders, but the slaps become punches and the hands are his instead of mine and I'm saying, "Why are you hitting me? Stop hitting me!"

I assert myself through defiance and learn to suck all the air out of a room with my fiery explosions while he becomes more and more of an island. My reaction to him being stronger is to become louder and more volatile. In the shadow of my outbursts, my brother is inadvertently ignored, seen by Mom and Dad as robust, buoyant, and strong. But in time his own anger boils over and he begins to assert himself with an equal volatility. Now I have a bloody nose while he's storming out of the rooms and slamming old Victorian doors on loose hinges, momentarily made visible by his rage. To be seen is to be loved, even if it means throwing a punch.

An Austrian named Sigmund Freud says the reason I have a fat lip is because of the Oedipus complex, which is named after a Greek fellow who killed his father and married his mother. He says that my brother and I are fighting for Mom's attention. It tracks even though she understandably feels like she has no more attention to give. Another Austrian fellow named Alfred Adler says that I have a bloody nose because of the order in which my brother and I were born. A British guy named John Bowlby says my black eye has something to do with attachment theory and it's all about the bonds we made with Mom and Dad as infants.

But they're all just theories and the why is less important than the what. Anger is the what. White-hot rage. The exact mechanisms of why only matter if they can be corrected. But we're ticking all the boxes of "happy family" and "good parenting," so no one really understands *why* my knuckles are bruised and everyone is mad.

History is full of fraternal chaos: Romulus and Remus, Thor and Loki, Cain and Abel. It's as if brothers are mythologically destined to clash. And because we're boys, Dad sees the blows, tears, bruises, and blood as an exercise in resilience. He says I need a "thicker skin." Dad's intended lesson is that the world is full of hard knocks and it's important to learn how to take a punch. He's not wrong.

But my skin isn't getting thicker. It's getting thinner. Instead of making me stronger, the escalating eruptions of violence are tearing away at everything inside of me. I feel my mind begin to drift away from my body with no way to step back in. And because the real source of it all is not one thing but many, it's impossible to really understand. My brother points his ire at me and becomes what the *DSM* calls an inescapable stress, and my brain and his brain and everyone's brain start to flood with stress hormones that none of us can pronounce. All any of us want is to feel safe and everyone is asking the same questions without daring to say them out loud. Did I cause this? Is this my fault?

Doug assures Mom and me that this isn't about fault or blame, but the words are forgotten before we leave the office. He suggests I try simply saying "Okay" when I feel my defiance surging. I promise I'll try and follow Mom back to the elevator. But saying "Okay" isn't enough. The little Dutch boy only had ten fingers and as per the calculations I made with Dad, this levee has eleven holes. The elevator door closes and I feel the bottom drop.

4

It's not that I'm smart, it's just that

I stay with problems longer.

—Albert Einstein

In fifth grade I test into the Extended Learning Program (ELP), which is an extension of the general classroom curriculum in Utah schools. The program aims to "meet the needs of identified gifted/talented and high ability students" through "skill development with higher order thinking skills in both critical and creative thinking." My brother tested into the program two years ago and now, despite a slow unraveling at home, we're both "gifted." At the very least, I'm smart enough to exhaust anyone who might argue with me.

The ELP teacher, Ms. Mathis, shows our class a black-and-white photo of an old man with long, thinning gray hair, kind eyes, and what looks like a very long tongue, and we laugh. We all know who Albert Einstein is and we know he was very smart. She tells our class that matter and energy are interchangeable. $E = mc^2$. The energy of anything is equal to its mass multiplied by the speed of light squared. She also tells us that the whole universe consists of *only* matter and energy and lots of space, and that atoms make up everything.

My ten-year-old mind likes the idea that everything everywhere is all the same stuff, just moving at different speeds. Some-how, it makes sense. I raise my hand to be sure I understand and ask if my desk is just energy slowed down and she answers, "Ac-cording to Einstein, yes. Everything." She continues to amaze me when she says that my body is 99.9999999 percent space and I wonder how something so solid can be so empty inside.

As I trudge home, I become increasingly unsettled by this theory of everything. I mash my thumb and forefinger together and marvel that there is in fact space between them and every-thing else. As concrete as the world seems, it's more empty than full. The pavement is apparently the same thing as the chestnut tree. Which is the same as the cracked sidewalk I use for a bike jump. Which is the same as the aluminum slats pulled askew in the window of the apartment building with cracked, white paint. And the plums smashed across the concrete. And the green grass. And the Victorian bricks. And the screen door slamming behind me. And my dad, sitting in front of me, correcting papers with a red pen, slashing across some poor student's test . . . it's all the same. Before saying hi, I ask, "If $E = mc^2$ and I am more space than matter, does anything *matter* at all?"

"Jeeeeeezus! Welcome home, Cor Por!" he laughs.

"If everything is the same thing, then does anything matter?" I insist. He caps his pen, pauses, and finally says, "Well, I suppose it's the way it's all arranged that gives it meaning . . . it's how it's put together. But then again, in the grand scheme of things . . . no, it probably doesn't matter in the way we think it does."

In sixth grade, I take another test to determine if I'll skip regular middle school and take advanced classes at West High where Dad teaches. I know that I can think because I think *a lot,* but I don't know if I'm "smart" in the way that the other students are. Two years ago, my brother took the test and skipped middle school and

I worry if I don't pass I'll be branded with the most horrifying label of all: normal. I'm relieved when the results come back.

On the first day of seventh grade I confidently pour a cup of coffee in one of Dad's thick plastic mugs. I hate the taste, but Mom and Dad do it and my brother does it too, so I do it to be like them.

Dad starts the rusty Suburban with a roar. The fan belt squeals while my brother takes his rightful seat in front, and I realize that I'm interrupting a ritual. For two years, they've been driving to school together and suddenly I feel like an outsider in a sacred space. I'm a boy sitting behind two men who sip their coffee and listen to the measured tones of NPR. My mouth is dry with anxiety, so I keep sucking back the milky fluid, which I've sweetened with enough sugar to give an elephant diabetes.

My brother is fourteen now and his voice has dropped. His eyes are darker and his arms bigger. The two years between us seem monstrous and I'm suddenly horrified about being twelve years old in school with eighteen-year-olds. Is being smart worth this gut-twisting anxiety? Why am I sweating? I need to shit. I think I might die from all the nerves and begin to shake. Maybe drinking more coffee will help.

Thankfully, the awkwardness of puberty makes just about anything a reason to bond. Currently, I'm a hippie because my brother is. This particular brand of teenage rebellion is called "granola." My clothes are a tribal calling card and I wear tie-dyed shirts with dancing bears and skulls wrapped in roses. My hair is growing long, my nose is too big, I have zits and braces, and have moved on from Guns N' Roses to the Grateful Dead and Bob Dylan. I make friends with other gangly teens only because we listen to the same bands. Our music is chosen less from taste than belonging. We split headphones one ear apiece, and Dylan sings:

> "I came in from the wilderness, a creature void of form
> Come in, she said, I'll give you shelter from the storm"

Above all, I love my visual arts course, which is taught by a balding man with a thinning ponytail that's often tied in a bun. The free flow of his class is natural to me. It's a meritocracy where distinction is measured not by stature but by the time invested and quality of work produced. In other words, it doesn't matter that I'm short and skinny and my wool socks and high-top hiking boots make my legs look like sticks. Here, I shine. These hours narrow my focus and my mind is no longer fragmented, but singular. Art is a gift that never stops giving. It's un-wanting even though it commands attention, and it's one of two things that I know to be truly altruistic. The other is nature.

Nature is the only other reprieve I get from my hyperactive brain. On the weekends we all climb into the Suburban in darkness and drive icy roads to Alta. Along the way we collect a cadre of scraggly dentists and lawyers who keep part-time jobs as ski patrollers on the weekends, clinging to youth and skiing for free. They have messy hair and stubble and bowed tan lines from where their ski goggles sit. Mom turns around and reminds us to put on our sunscreen.

She's the only woman in the car and sits opposite Dad on the bench seat and touches his leg while he makes filthy jokes. My brother and I are stuffed in the back listening to music. I have a beautiful yellow Sony Sports Walkman with lots of gray buttons and a small LCD screen that sheds just enough light for me to read the lyrics on the cassette fold-outs.

Once at Alta, we're released into the wild and rarely fight. There's no time for it. From the moment we park to the moment the fan belt squeals at the end of the day I chase my brother, both of us laying deep arcs in the snow with the edges of our skis. Here value is measured in skill and speed and the ability to throw our rubbery bodies off higher and higher cliffs. Here there is no time for thoughts because we're already going too fast. That's what happens when learning to ski overlaps with learning to walk. At 50 mph, you can feel every crystal and undulation in the snow and there's no time to consider anything but the next turn and how to avoid splatting against a tree. These days of cold wind and the silence of snowfall are magical and complete. They're another gift that gives pause to the accelerating family freefall of the weeks. But Mondays always come.

My brother chases me up the stairs in a rage. I cower in the fetal position on the carpet as violent white flashes pulse behind my eyes. His fist crashes against my temple again and again until Dad manages to pull him off. Mom stands at the top of the stairs and screams as I wipe blood from my lip. I spit at him over Dad and it lands in his hair. He swings and misses while Mom screams "*Stop!*" and the room is still for a moment. He's a better fighter. Bigger. Stronger. Faster. No matter how badly I want to fight back, it just isn't in me and I always end up on the ground. These days it seems to happen every night.

With Dad between us and Mom watching, I have no outlet other than a scream. I double over and push all the air from my lungs until it's silent. But it's not enough. I stand, look at everyone, and kick my foot through a thick window, channeling all the rage into an explosion of glass. A small cut on my ankle leaks blood and I notice thousands of tiny shards reflecting from the carpet like little stars. These emotions are not directional but more like the big bang. They are the energy of rage and love. They are the hard matter of fists and embraces. They are the expanding space between us all.

By the end of seventh grade, I'm feeling more distant as the space inside me grasps at the final .000001 percent it hasn't yet claimed.

I'm depressed and my grades are slipping. I discover the over-whelming joy of skipping school and huddling in alleys with older kids, smoking cigarettes and drinking, which I have no idea are tied to the rage of home.

Harvard psychiatrist Dr. Judith Lewis Herman, who studies the mechanisms and results of trauma, contends that the majority of *all* psychiatric diagnosis is really just Complex Post-traumatic Stress. That assertion will be supported when Kaiser and the Centers for Disease Control and Prevention (CDC) explore the seas of developmental trauma and toxic stress as they relate to "later-life health and wellbeing." Specifically, the study explores the occurrence of Adverse Childhood Experiences, or ACEs.

Looking at experiences that occur between birth and age seventeen, a Kaiser/CDC study categorized different kinds of abuse and neglect that are understood to produce toxic stress. Individuals are scored on the ACEs measure, a simple 0–10 tally corresponding to the number of adverse experiences endured. The study tracked participants' health through their lives and found that stress is *literally* toxic.

The questionnaire is distilled to ten simple questions.

Before your 18th birthday, did a parent or other adult in the household often or very often swear at you, insult you, put you down, or humiliate you or act in a way that made you afraid that you might be physically hurt?

If you answer yes, your ACE score is 1. And if you have one adverse childhood experience, the chances you have two or more are 87 percent. Sixty-two to 64 percent of adults have at least one.

Next question:

Before your 18th birthday, did a parent or other adult in the house-
hold often or very often push, grab, slap, or throw something at
you? Or ever hit you so hard that you had marks or were injured?

Yes? Your ACE score is 2. And so on. As a person's ACE score
increases, so does the likelihood of a host of health issues, including but not limited to depression, ADHD, bipolar disorder,
severe obesity, diabetes, heart disease, cancer, stroke, chronic ob-
structive pulmonary disease, broken bones, and sexually trans-
mitted infections (thanks, Lisa; you did say I'd never forget you).
People with an ACE score of 4 or higher are twice as likely to be
smokers and *seven times* more likely to be alcoholic. Had enough
yet? An ACE score of four or higher increases the risk of conditions like chronic bronchitis and emphysema by nearly 400 percent and attempted suicide by 1,200 percent. Individuals with
high ACE scores are more likely to be violent, more likely to
miss work, more likely to have financial problems, more likely to
experience the end of a marriage, and more likely to endure abusive relationships. ACE score of 6 or higher? Your life span is at
risk of being reduced by as much as *twenty* years.

I have an ACE score of 4.

It's May now and every night ends the same. A fight erupts in
the kitchen or in the driveway or on the lawn. The stress is palpable and tastes like burnt coffee, with the same nauseating jit-
ters, sweat, anxiety, and the overwhelming urge to shit because
our insides are exploding.

The violence and chaos build with every blow until eventually
one punch is thrown that extinguishes the light of childhood and
changes our family forever. Time stops as the front door slams

and the doorbell hums into a silence that will last decades. Mom looks at me and whispers, "Are you okay?" but I can't tell if she's asking me or herself. I want to be innocent in this violence but I am not. I'm just better at hiding my part. Mom moves aside and stares at Dad. I walk upstairs, close my bedroom door, and shake.

The rest of the night has no edges and the world seems smudged. If I didn't exist, would this house be the same? Am I cause or effect? Would everything be better if I just dissolved?

For my brother and me, abuse is two-sided. But because I'm the one who ends up bleeding, it's easy to overlook my culpability. What I know is that for us, conflict is a catalyst for attention. We don't need a reason to fight because the fight itself has become the reason. In that way, getting the shit kicked out of me is just another means to feel cared for. The fight is the shortcut to the attention we crave as we seesaw back and forth between violence and victim, using both sides to claw for love. How it got this way is anyone's guess. Blame is useless amidst madness. But it's clear to me that I co-author this chaos.

5

There is no greater agony than bearing

an untold story inside you.

—Maya Angelou

Halfway through eighth grade my grades have fallen so far that Mom and Dad are worried I'll be expelled. Dad gets updates from my teachers on which classes I've missed, which is most of them. Sometimes he comes by to see if I'm there at all. I have insomnia and the days have become a lethargic march. Unable to keep my eyes open in school, I skip more classes because I have a new identity. Now I am a grunge thug and wear flannel.

My jeans are baggy and dirty, and my hair is long. I've been on Prozac for a year but have expanded my range and do LSD for the first time in a friend's basement. We listen to *Nirvana Unplugged* on vinyl for eight hours straight, dragging our fingers through the carpet and across the walls while the world shines, shimmers, ripples, and changes color, and Kurt Cobain sings: "All in all is all we are / All in all is all we are."

Every time I smoke weed, I black out and have a four-hour panic attack. Art class is the last vestige of my education these days and I often go high. But today I've overdone it and forget where I am. When my teacher asks, "Cory, are you okay?" I have the sense of waking up having never been asleep. I can't tell if I'm speaking or thinking and don't know if I ever answer but am certain my eyes say enough. I hate this feeling but keep smoking in a masochistic search for approval.

On one of the first warm days of spring, I share a joint laced with PCP. The world washes over me like toppling waves as I float in and out of consciousness. The lack of control is horrifying and I promise myself I'll never smoke again. From now on, I'll only pretend to inhale but rarely will. I'll be an imposter and add a new layer to the Russian doll that is me.

Home is more chaos than calm and my parents ask if I'd like to go away for the summer. I wonder why I need to leave instead of my brother. The message is murky: Am I the issue, or is he? I think it's him and he thinks it's me, but it's *us*. All of us. They're looking for a solution to the crisis and this is the best they have. But the heart rarely understands logic and I leave, feeling like the problem. For now, resolution comes from my absence.

I start ninth grade at Judge Memorial Catholic High School. I wear pressed white shirts, khaki pants, and knit ties that feel cheap. Private school means more rules and guardrails that we all hope might keep me in line.

No drugs of any kind.
No T-shirts (under our button-ups) depicting alcohol, drugs, or inappropriate language.
All students must take theology class and attend chapel.
Hair is to be clean and combed, and long hair on boys is tolerated but discouraged.
Attendance must be 95 percent or higher.
Believe in God.
If you don't, pretend.
Etc. etc. etc.

In theology class, I'm required to memorize and recite the books of the Bible in order. I consider myself an atheist because that's what Dad calls himself, but I'm fascinated by biblical stories of vengeance and brothers murdering brothers. The Bible is chock-full of infanticide, which seems an odd choice for a loving God. Children are cast into exile and whole lineages are smitten in a single breath. In the Bible, everyone comes from a fucked-up family.

There's no art class, so I pour myself into English and read Huxley, Homer, and Harper Lee. Dickens and Salinger, and some Shakespeare. It's a clichéd collection, but one that begins to open my mind in a new way. Reading is no longer a chore as I travel seamlessly from past to future. Literature connects me to a world outside of myself and I'm less alone. Just as with art, my mind narrows and the world is quiet. Books are a reservoir of emotion and a place to go when I'm trying to make sense of everything, which is always. All words are borrowed. The beauty of writing is how they flow through us and arrange themselves as something new but familiar. We can be unique and belong at the same time. In moments of confusion, anger, and sadness, words lend comfort, letting us know that someone else has navigated the same tempestuous tides and survived.

I'm standing in front of the entire ninth-grade class with three pages of meticulous cursive that looks just like Mom's. There is a pond of shadowed faces staring at me and my knees are weak, which has nothing to do with being onstage but everything to do with what I'm about to read. I clear my throat.

A Day in the Life

by Cory Richards

Every day begins the same. I roll from bed and pass my fingers through my matted hair and hide the bottle from the night before.

Exhaling into my hand, I retch from the smell of my breath. Jameson and sleep. This is me, again, raw and uncensored.

There are giggles and gasps as teachers shoot to attention and shift. Everyone is staring and leaning in and I can hear their chairs squeak. I keep reading. *It's not that I don't know it's wrong, it's just that I don't care.* Now the adults are shooting glances back and forth, but no one's stopping me. It's not because the writing is good but because they're as riveted and curious as the students. I read the last line: *I look in the mirror, tired of my own face.* I'm in the dean's office three minutes later and she's on the phone with Mom.

I try to explain that this was fiction and quote Virginia Woolf from my English class as evidence: "Lies will flow from my lips, but there may perhaps be some truth mixed up with them; it is for you to seek out this truth and decide whether any part of it is worth keeping." It's the only class I'm getting a good grade in.

The dean is shocked for a moment before rolling her eyes. It's a good argument. Mom shrugs, exasperated and familiar with my ability to pull random quotes from the air to support my arguments. It was all made up aside from my hair being matted and the part about my face, but now I'm peeing in a cup. The drug test is negative, but I'm asked politely to leave Judge forever and I remember the priest in chapel saying something about "one bad apple."

I know *what* I'm fighting but I have no idea what I'm fighting *for* other than my emancipation from childhood. At some point every generation is lost. We must be. How else can we find ourselves?

Back in public school, I'm unbound. No one's checking my attendance, so I just stop going and edge toward dropping out. For two parents in education, it's a tragedy. I'm fourteen years old and will wear my rebellion with pride for twenty years until I share a stage with an Afghan woman as she tells her story of disguising herself as a boy and walking for hours a day to school in Taliban-ruled Afghanistan. She was willing to die for an education.

But while she's half a world away risking her life, I do acid in the park. Rather than the LSD generating curiosity and connection, my mind goes sideways and I'm convinced that my insides are fluid. If I lie down, they'll spill out of me like an orange Slurpee. It's fun until it turns on me and nothing is sparkly at all. I run my fingers through the grass and try to hold on. I squeeze harder but it just pulls out with a crunch and everyone is laughing but I can't hear them. I'm far away now and the sky is clear but gray and the trees are losing their leaves and everything has lost its color. I close my eyes and pray to a God I've never known to make everything just stop.

This is one of my last days of freedom but there is no freedom to it because I'm trapped inside a ceaseless mind that is mine but feels controlled by something else entirely.

6

Be silent and listen: have you recognized

your madness and do you admit it?

—C. G. Jung

I stand alone in the darkness of the family den, surrounded by the shapes of my parents after they've left the room. A pen sits on a stack of half-graded papers that finally sent Dad to bed. The dial-up modem blinks green, casting a momentary shadow of a nest of wires. Dark mounds of overstuffed furniture with delicate floral upholstery are silhouetted against tall windows that frame the fireplace that Santa Claus used until I was eight. An array of glass vases sits on the mantel, throwing distorted shadows that look like water.

I sit at the computer and lay my head on the keyboard. It feels soft and sticky against my cheek as my legs bounce. The chair gently swivels and I look for sleep even though it feels as if I've forgotten how. Eventually the gentle hum of the computer becomes so overwhelming that I'm forced to move.

The darkness feels soupy as I walk to the back door and stare at the driveway. All I can see are the black arms of the peach tree and the shapes of blossoms that will become the fruit that will fall to the pavement and rot in the August heat, leaving sticky dark stains that remind me of a peach crime scene.

I'm shocked to feel tears as my brain begins to race, swirling in a whirlpool of thought that topples over itself. My mind is always fast, but this feels very different. The words and colors and sounds become a single, encompassing hum until eventually it all distills into a loud, pulsing sensation. It's my own heart, beating in sync with bright flashes of white behind my eyes. My head feels disconnected from my body and I'm somehow formless but trapped. I seem to float but am tethered. The hum loudens to a roar until it swallows anything rational and concrete.

I imagine myself being pulled apart by two freight trains speeding in opposite directions, torn between sanity and something else . . . something frightening. The noise in my head and the silence surrounding me warps, bends, and drones as my hands cover my ears and I pull at my hair. Like waking up, the horrifying reality of madness appears to me slowly and all at once, and I wish to die because all I want is for the noise to stop.

For days I tell no one and hope that hiding it will make it disappear. I've heard my madness but don't want to admit it. I'll learn later that this is my rite of passage into the world of bipolar disorder (BD). It's my first "mixed episode," when hypomania and crushing depression overlap. I'm initiated. Madness lives in me.

Primary Children's psychiatric unit sits at the end of an impossibly long hallway of hard, blue-gray carpet. The walls are blank slates of eggshell white. Or khaki. Or pewter. Some neutral color easily painted over. The hall is wide enough to tackle, restrain, and quiet any screams before they reach the ears of children whose sicknesses you *can* see. The desolate, cold corridor is my induction into institutionalized life. There are no plants and no art and the only two things that calm my mind are gone.

I smell Band-Aids and tissues and adolescent hormones mixed with the burning smell of a tired vacuum. It's one of the most distinct odors of my life and it hangs in the back of my nostrils for decades. The steel doors close behind me and I hear the unique heavy *clunk* of magnetic locks. It's a sound I've never heard and will never forget and I wonder how something so simple can imprint itself in memory so completely, the way a hot stove does the first and only time you make the mistake of reaching for the red coils.

Mom checks me in and I slouch low with my legs splayed in ripped jeans, defiant and exhausted. I feel loose in my skin. My face is pale, drawn, and greasy, with dark circles under my eyes from the nights I no longer sleep. I sit in an upholstered chair with a faint trail of mucus smeared across the armrest and stare.

After a few minutes, a therapist with a puffy face framed by straight, jet-black hair invites me into her office. She wears an emerald blouse layered under a cardigan and offers me a chair while Enya plays through the air conditioner.

"Nice to meet you, Courtney."

"It's Cory."

"So what brings you here, Cory?"

"I don't feel good. I'm depressed."

"Who told you that you were depressed and how long have you been feeling this way?" She stares.

Depression erases the memory of not being depressed. I feel everything too deeply, so I've given up feeling at all. I know I haven't always felt this way but can't remember when or under what circumstances that's ever been the case. It's like asking someone to recall an alternate reality. I finally answer, "I guess I just don't remember it another way."

"Are you taking drugs, Cory?"

I don't answer.

"Would you like your mother to leave so we can talk?" This is a ruse. The absence of a parent makes you feel safer admitting your transgressions, but it's really just a game of telephone. You tell the therapist something and she relays the information to your parents with a clinical bent.

Mom stands to leave, shutting the door too gently on her way out. I turn back to the therapist and tell her everything by saying nothing.

"Cory, are you thinking about hurting yourself?"

I collapse on her desk and hide my face in my arms as my legs bounce. My cheeks feel wet against my skin and peel off as I lift my head enough to wipe my nose across my forearm.

I want refuge and death seems safe. I've thought of many ways to kill myself, but I don't know how. There are knives but that seems too slow and I don't really want to cut myself because it hurts too much. We don't have guns. Mom hates guns because her brother used one to end his own life. Anyway, that would be too messy. I've pulled all the pill bottles from the cabinet and wondered which I should take and how many but I don't know. I've slung a rope from the rafters in the garage and hung my whole weight on it by my neck, keeping my feet on the ground to abort because I was scared of what I would think if I stepped off a chair, suspended with no way down. I like the feeling of hanging and the way my eyes rhythmically bulge with my pulse. But it's not that I want to die. It's that living feels too confusing. They say suicide is irrational. In some moments, though, it seems the most rational thing of all. I don't tell the therapist any of this.

She invites Mom back in and says, "I think Cory could really benefit from a short stay with us, just to get his medications straightened out and restore some balance at home. Unfortunately, we don't have any space at the moment, so you'll have to wait until a bed opens up."

Relief washes over me because as bad as things are, being locked away in a psychiatric ward feels extreme, and the idea of being left here is suffocating. The smell bothers me. Enya bothers me. The therapist's emerald blouse bothers me. Everything makes me want to run, but I can tell Mom is disappointed. She wants me to stay.

We walk back through the office and around the semicircular counter and across the lobby. But before I can make it to the end of the desolate tunnel and into freedom, a short bald man rushes toward us and I am suspended. The lights hum and flicker and he says, "Mrs. Richards?"

"Yes, are you Ivan?" I wonder how she knows his name.

"I am. I'm so glad I caught you. We've just had a bed open. Shall we do the intake?" He speaks with a smile I instinctively hate.

Before Mom can respond my fist clenches and I watch it make contact with his face in slow motion. I smash his jaw and feel the crunch of his nose and teeth as blood flies everywhere and I begin to run. But the hallway is long and the alarm has been sounded. Large tattooed orderlies in white are chasing me, but I'm too fast, too agile, and far smarter than them. My shoulder hits the magnetic door, but I feel nothing as it gives way to the interior of the hospital, where I can weave through the doctors and nurses in blue scrubs holding manila folders. They stare at me with shock and awe. The orderlies' footsteps are heavy behind me and their keys are jangling and they're screaming for someone to stop me but no one dares because they see that I'm crazy. I leap over a railing and drop three stories and land like a superhero as the linoleum buckles under me and everyone is shocked because I'm so incredible. They realize that I'm no normal wayward teen and they cannot stop me. The main entrance is just ahead. I see sunlight and blue sky and use my incredible brain to break the locks on the doors before I even get there. Red sirens are spinning and the alarm is blaring as a burly security officer dives toward me. He misses as I leap sideways onto the wall and run in a horizontal arc over his head, defying gravity as he looks at me with awe. I'm free and running toward my merchant ship again.

"Oh, Ivan, thank God. Yes, please, let's do the intake," Mom says too quickly. His nose is not broken and there is no blood. I feel his hand grasp my forearm.

"What do you mean?" I ask.

"We'd like to keep you here for a few days, Courtney."

"It's Cory."

His bald head gleams and reflects a white spot from the fluorescent lights. My jaw tightens and I step toward the door, but Ivan pivots and steps in front. I look at him and then back to Mom.

"Did you know about this?" I ask.

"Sweetie, no. This is just . . ."

I stare, begging her to reconsider. She tucks her lips into each other and raises her eyebrows the way she does when she digs in. My meek appeal turns to rage and I swear at her.

"I'm going to need to ask you to calm down, Courtney."

"Fuck you too, *I-van*!" Even to my own ears, the language comes as a shock. "I'm not staying here!" I shout.

But Ivan is calm and unimpressed. "Courtney . . . Follow me, please. I don't want to have you escorted." I wonder if the tattooed orderlies are hiding just out of sight. Mom says nothing.

He leads us down another long hall to a corner room. The door is open and a dejected teenager is sitting on the edge of a bed mumbling to himself. The neckline of his T-shirt is stretched low. Faint yellow stains and smudges of dirt spot the chest. Surely I'm not as sick as him. He looks up at us, stands, and paces.

"Cory will be sharing your room tonight until we can find him a more suitable roommate." The boy says nothing. More suitable? It's clear that my new bunkmate is immersed in or recovering from a psychotic break and I'm scared. I want to run but I'm a superhero only in my brain and there is no merchant vessel in sight.

"I fucking hate you!" I spit. Mom cries quietly and inhales the way exhausted mothers do and turns to follow Ivan down the hall. I stand at the scene of my exile and stare blankly, looking up just in time to watch her turn the corner and disappear.

All I can feel is rage, seething and complete. But I don't hate her, I hate me. In my mother, I see myself. In her face. In her mannerisms. In her pain. She doesn't deserve any of what I offer in exchange for her love. But the problem with an unwell mind is that it makes you blind to the world. Through my own relentless drive to be seen, I've created a cage. It is at once my salvation and my despair and if I could take back all my words I would. But I can't.

I don't know if I sleep. My roommate talks to people that I can't see. He sleeps in his clothes and wrestles the sheets. I lie still and stare at the ceiling, trying not to breathe. I sleep in my clothes too because I don't want the sheets to touch me. When I wake up, my collar hangs stretched and low.

"Do you think you can do anything, Courtney?" a new therapist asks.

"It's Cory."

"Do you think you can do anything, Cory?" She's digging for delusions of grandeur and I know it.

"What do you mean?"

"Could you build a building in a day or perhaps fly? Do you ever hear voices, Cory?"

I hear yours, I think, and I want to rip your lips off. "Maybe whispers sometimes," I say—it's a dangerous way to answer. I don't want to be hearing voices and I've never had any auditory hallucinations. But I want to be sick enough that someone will care. Some piece of me is actually fighting to stay here. Whispers seems a reasonable gambit.

"Do they ever tell you to do things?"

"No." A yes here would be a step too far.

The inquiry persists for a tense hour of manipulation and mental acrobatics. At one point I hear one of the doctors say something about early-onset paranoid schizophrenia, but that's shortly laid to rest. Bipolar? Maybe? Yes, bipolar. That fits nicely.

The mid-1990s were banner years for bipolar diagnosis in troubled teens. Bipolar disorder, the artist formerly known as manic-depression, is expressed in extremes. Imagine the earth's equator as the midline of emotional expression. Most people live along or near that line. Bipolar people are explorers of the polar regions, often racing between them in no time at all.

Bipolar 1 and 2 are distinct diagnoses, and one is not more or less severe than the other, though type 1 is sometimes easier to identify. Both are manageable and both can be deadly.

I'm diagnosed with bipolar 2, which the doctors tell me describes "individuals who have had at least one major depressive episode and at least one hypomanic episode but have never experienced a manic episode." This leaves a lot of room for interpretation and I'm confused and ask, "What's the difference?"

Hypomania and mania are distinct but share similar and often overlapping symptoms. Racing thoughts. Reduced need for sleep. Exaggerated sense of self. Irritability. Impulsive decision-making. Distractibility. Obsessive rumination. Many of these symptoms are shared with ADHD as well, but mania is not. So here is a glimpse of what mania looks like:

I just punched a wall after not sleeping for three days but I'm fine, probably the best I've ever been because I'm starting six new projects that I'm sure will make me a billionaire, so I gambled my savings away to impress the neighbor's wife into sleeping with me after getting drunk and doing enough cocaine to kill a horse before calling a prostitute to come over and have some unprotected . . . oh look, a cat.

It's not always this bad, but it can be. That's why full-blown mania can be easier to spot.

Hypomania can express similarly, but it's less intense. In the absence of identifiable mania, a hypomanic person can appear to be exceptionally high-functioning, wildly creative, charming, and enviably social. For me, it's big ideas, racing thoughts, electric lust, and an almost incomprehensible distractibility balanced by unbreakable focus and the requisite irritability: if you dare interrupt my fixation, the furniture best be nailed to the floor.

The origins of BD are complicated. Children born to parents who have it are far more likely to develop the disorder but aren't necessarily predisposed to it. Genetics and epigenetics usually play a role, but it's not clear exactly how much.

Robust psychological studies clearly show that childhood trauma is a strong risk factor for psychiatric disorders and multiple traumas are more frequent in patients with BD. The correlations between trauma and people who suffer from BD are simply too strong to ignore. Among the types of trauma (emotional, physical, and sexual), only emotional abuse has a suggested dose effect with BD. In essence, more emotional abuse leads to greater risk. Then again, trauma doesn't always lead to BD, but people who are diagnosed are far more likely to have endured a traumatic childhood. So even though 80 percent of individuals with BD have a family history of the disorder, it's too reductive to say that people are born with it.

It's vital to understand that BD is not handed off like a drunken kiss that lands you with angry cold sores for the rest of your life. It seems to develop over time, most commonly in the teens or early twenties. The monster erupts from a murky sea of DNA struck by the lightning of lived experience. Too many factors are present to lay the blame neatly at the feet of any single event or person.

Based on the numbers, it's likely that one of my parents has suffered from undiagnosed BD. Who knows. As for me, I'm still not sure what hormone-driven adolescent could *not* be considered bipolar. But for now that's what they call me and what I'll call myself for many years. It's point, set, match. I'm officially "sick" and they give me new pills. These ones are pink and blue.

7

Once you went outlaw, then you were there,

and that's where you stayed.

—Alexandra Fuller, *Quiet Until the Thaw*

After a week of trying to wash the burned antiseptic smell from my nostrils, two big teenagers walk through the door of my room. One of them is named Barnes and I guess his weight at over 220 pounds. He grew up on a dairy farm and shows me later how he can rip a phone book in half. I don't remember the other's name, but he's shorter and wider.

Barnes and Shorter-than-Barnes are here to escort me from the psychiatric unit to a white van waiting downstairs. STB makes an effort to make me laugh and put me at ease while Barnes holds my arm with a farmboy grip and I don't feel at ease at all. I'm labeled as "high flight risk" and I assume that if I try to run their instructions are to sit on me.

I'm being moved from the hospital to a new home for broken kids called LifeLine for Youth, which is a hybrid inpatient-outpatient behavioral rehab program for kids with stretched collars and tired eyes. The tag line reads "When Good Kids Make Bad Decisions." The sliding door slams behind me and locks.

The white van turns left on South Temple and heads west past

Reservoir Park and I stare through the tinted glass, looking for my friends and freedom.

The van drives north past West High School and I see my dad's Suburban parked in its usual spot and look up to his classroom window on the fourth floor. I imagine his unintelligible handwriting slashing numbers across the whiteboard in frantic equations and wonder if this was part of his calculus when I was born. Does he know where I am? Can he feel me as I pass by? Does he know where they're taking me?

We turn left on West Center Street past Big West Oil, where flames punch from the top of skinny chimneys above a mess of piping. I don't look for anyone I know.

The white van parks.

The structure is a squat brick building surrounded on two sides by an irrigation ditch that doubles as a moat. It's the kind of architecture that tells you whatever you're here to do, it's going to suck—like going to the DMV or municipal court. Every spring, the reeds and grass that edge the water grow tall and beautiful and it's almost serene. But as the heat of the summer sets in, the foliage browns and the water stagnates and the whole area smells like decay. It's the smell of tadpoles and frogs and small fish rotting in the heat. Many things die here.

Tall, narrow windows set back behind brick pillars appear black from the exterior. But when you're looking out, it's the same purple hue with trapped air bubbles that all therapists' offices have and I wonder why they hate light so much. Inside, the windows cast long rectangles of muted sun that travel slowly across the tired carpet, expanding and contracting as the earth spins. They are reverse sundials. But for those of us kept here, time is suspended, uprooted from youth and planted in a blue chair.

Barnes and STB parade me through the front door and into a small office that's hot and yellow like an old photograph. They tell me that they've both been here for several months and are on "fourth phase," which affords them certain privileges like going back to school, running errands, and escorting new intakes from hospitals. "What's first phase?" I ask.

They take my shoes and belt because no one wants me to run away or hang myself. They explain that there are five phases and I'm a newcomer, so I'm on first phase. Second phase or higher makes me an "oldcomer." But all new intakes are referred to as "belt loops" because we're not allowed to move anywhere without an oldcomer holding the back of our pants, wrapping a thumb and forefinger through a belt loop. Belt loop newcomers look like zombies being driven from behind in some demeaning parade. Even standing in the urinal, there's a hand down the back of our pants and the only break is when we take a shit. As far as I can see the oldcomers are part of a despotic hierarchy of the blind leading the blind and I resent their smug superiority.

The bathrooms smell like urinal cakes and the lunchroom is an old greenhouse that's always stuffy and hot. The group room, the nucleus of LifeLine, is a large open space with gray carpet and a 10-foot-high drop ceiling that looks like an office building with industrial fluorescent lights. Twelve chunky white frames hang on a central wall, each emblazoned with one of the twelve steps of recovery as a road map to wellness. The thick black lines are imperfect because they've been stenciled in someone's garage and steps three, seven, and nine are crooked. Sixty blue plastic chairs are placed in arching lines that face the placards and the semicircle is bisected to create the "girls' side" and the "guys' side" so no one can give or receive covert hand jobs.

The group room seems well kept at first glance. But the place has scars and it's amazing what you can see when you sit in a chair for eight hours a day. There's a handful of repaired holes at fist and foot height. I see a sheen of mucus that someone wiped on the wall as they cried. A water-stained ceiling tile sits askew and peeks into darkness, cracked by a flying shoe when an old-comer was demoted back to first phase. Uneven holes in the window laminate create tiny glowing windows where the sun peeks through, peeled away as some kid was picked apart. I see a deep dent in the drywall where someone threw a chair.

Every group session is punctuated by joining hands and asking God to grant us serenity: *Grant me the serenity to accept this prison, the restraint to not curb you, and wisdom of some sort, but I don't know what.*

We say: "It works if you work it, so work it, you're worth it!" like a sullen cheer squad and add an a capella "Looooooooove ya, group!" with the same awkwardness as singing "Happy Birthday" at someone.

At the end of each eleven-hour day, a parade of cars lines up and oldcomers take newcomers back to their homes, where we eat and write moral inventories. As per the guidelines of the program, we sleep in rooms with nothing but mattresses and blankets on the floor. I think there must be some wildly misguided logic at play as well as an insurance nightmare waiting to happen because the rooms are locked from the outside and the windows can't be opened. God forbid there's a fire because we'll all die horrible deaths as we're consumed by flames. We'll have to be identified by our teeth and our parents will weep and regret every decision they ever made. I pray for a fire.

After two weeks they give me my shoes back but they still don't want me to hang myself, so they keep my laces and belt. At medication time, I'm given my pills in a paper shot glass and a Dixie cup of water that tastes like wax. I'm asked to lift my tongue to show them that I've swallowed, and they ask, "How are you feeling?" I shrug.

The real problem is I don't *feel* much of anything. A heavy chemical blanket has been laid over the anger, but it feels like I'm being told to go to sleep and that everything will be better when I wake up in thirty years. I feel hollow and try to fill it all up with food. I gain weight and stare through glassy eyes and sleep under the table during school until they reduce my dose. I'm quiet and withdrawn. Doing anything is impossible because just *being* is taking up all my effort.

After a few weeks I begin to scratch shallow gouges into my wrists and forearms and am fascinated by the sting. They make me clip my nails but I just scratch harder, peeling back the scabs until I bleed. The wounds are an attempt to externalize pain. Maybe if someone can just see it, they'll understand.

All the adults tell me to *fake it 'til I make it*, so I reluctantly start talking in group. When I'm feeling particularly vulnerable, my contributions are very genuine because I actually want out of this cycle. But usually I argue with the head therapist.

"You don't know anything about me!"

"I know enough," he replies.

I despise his goatee and wire-framed glasses and the way he has no neck from lifting weights. I hate his neatly buttoned shirt and pleated Dockers. I tell him that I could leave today and be just fine. I tell him that this is all fucking me up more than I already am.

"If you left today, you'd end up fucked up and on the street. You'd be another addict. You're not special, Cory." His reply is scathing. They call this tough love.

"Fuck you."

In 1963, psychologist Bob Rosenthal had an idea. He built a maze and got some rodents and then randomly labeled each rat as "maze bright" or "maze dull." His students were then assigned as caretakers of a rat that they already assumed had been identified as smart or dumb when in fact they were all just rats who liked food and water and maybe a gentle pat on the head. Not one had ever been tested in a maze.

Dr. Rosenthal's hypothesis was that people can and do unconsciously influence the performance of others simply through what we think of them. His students began running their respective rats through a series of basic tests like finding cheese at the end of a maze. Over time, the arbitrarily labeled "maze bright" rats did nearly twice as well as their counterparts on all tests performed. They were faster and more creative through the maze. This suggested that the students' unconscious bias toward the rats that were labeled "bright" affected every interaction between student and rodent: the way they held them, the way they spoke to them, the way they fed them. Through unconscious bias, the "smart" rats—who were no different from the "dumb" rats—had magically become "smart" rats.

When he applied a similar test to children, the results were the same. After all the children were given an IQ test, a handful of them were selected at random and labeled "academic bloomers." Their test scores had not been considered and there was no evidence to support that any of the chosen children were in fact brighter than the others. After a year, during which the researchers observed teacher-student interactions, a second IQ test was given. The bloomers had blossomed while the control group had shown no marked shift. Some challenged Rosenthal's conclusions as dubious, but over time the results were replicated in every area from leadership to athletics. What we think of someone affects how we treat them, and they shape themselves into that image through osmosis.

Rosenthal's experiments demonstrate what's known as the Pygmalion effect: Higher expectations lead to greater performance. It isn't always about the underlying intellectual acuity or talent of an individual; it's also about how they are treated. Of course, there are outliers and people who are actually born with greater and lesser degrees of talent or intellect. Also, expectation can go too far if too much pressure is applied. But what the study proved is that if you're treated as though you're smart, you often get smarter. Because the educators *thought* certain kids were brighter, they unknowingly provided more personal feedback, sat the "gifted" students closer to the chalkboard, were kinder and more patient, were more approving in general, and even smiled more often. They also thought that they were unbiased. Convinced, even.

The inverse is also true. If someone thinks you're a fucking problem, an addict, a fuck-up, and broken, they're going to treat you differently despite all their best intentions otherwise, which can foster a slow, steady reduction, stripping away confidence and self-love until it all becomes a repeated, entrenched story. The irony is that this contraction often occurs in the care of those who are genuinely trying to help.

The so-called troubled-teen industry is also big business. In 2021, twenty-six years from now, the American Bar Association will report that the industry receives $23 billion annually in public funds. Many of the facilities are run for profit and receive enormous sums from Medicaid, Medicare, and other government and private sources. Well intentioned as some of this treatment may be, it has one glaring blind spot.

As a general rule, kids don't fly off the handle in a vacuum. While abuse, trauma, and toxic stress aren't exclusively products of home life, they're often born there. Sending kids away only to have them return to the same situation and then expecting them to stay healthy is like treating someone for burn wounds, only to ask them to walk back into a house fire. When toxic influences come from outside sources, they're often ignored or swept under the rug of the child's behavior. Regardless of where the abuse comes from, often the child won't speak about it out of fear that they won't be believed. Or worse, they think it *is* actually *all* their fault. By way of the Pygmalion effect, those beliefs are reinforced.

Ironically, I've been treated as "maze bright" *and* "maze dull." In fact, the two characterizations rely on each other. I've demonstrated an inclination toward high achievement, been seated toward the front of the class, and have been smiled at. But now I've plunged off an invisible edge and the fall has been spectacular and swift. That I was so "good" amplifies the idea that now I'm "bad." Everyone is confused and Mom and Dad and the therapists are trying to answer everyone's questions about what's happened. They are looking for a digestible reason or a truth that can explain everything. I wish there was just one thing to trace it back to and I look for a singular incident, straining to remember some defining moment that never happened. The only event is life itself.

8

Fuck you I won't do what you tell me!

—Rage Against the Machine

I've been at LifeLine for two months and am on second phase. I bring newcomers home with me every night and we sleep in my old bedroom, which is now just a pile of sheets and mattresses. Tonight, Mom serves us Thai peanut chicken over heaps of white rice. I love the thick sauce, which is just coconut milk and an acre's worth of chunky peanut butter. This meal shows the depth of her sacrifice because she hates coconut and loathes peanuts in anything. It's a hopeful window of calm.

But tonight I want to run.

They call it "copping out" and it's the surest way to undo any progress I've made. I've watched kids disappear only to return tattered, defiant, and defeated. It can be a day or three weeks, but they always come back with stretched necklines. I haven't even considered running away until I'm sitting in front of the chicken.

I've always been two people and each has a million different moods. I am my own merchant vessel commanded by two captains. One is mild-mannered and measured and searches for smooth seas. The other is a mischievous trickster who longs for big waves and storms. He loves being drenched and cold and starving and craves adventure, always searching for the edge of the map. He's also a selfish sailor and only relinquishes control once the mast is broken and we're adrift. It's frustrating, but I need both of me because, as Franklin D. Roosevelt pointed out, drawing on an old saying, "a smooth sea never made a good sailor."

I'll never know why or how they trade places in the boat. We all have a darker passenger; it just feels like mine dictates my decisions more often and I'm all too willing when he takes control. Tonight I stare at my plate and watch myself shift at the helm. I take one last bite of chicken and sail into a storm.

I ask to use the bathroom and slip out the front door and run into the darkness, unsure of where I'm going or why or what will happen. I figure I have five minutes to put as much distance between the house and me before someone says, "Cory's taking an awfully long shit," and everything explodes into chaos. But I have adrenaline and hot summer air and freedom on my side, and for a moment, I feel manically liberated. I know if they catch me, they'll take my shoes and belt and someone will have their hand in the back of my pants again. But they won't find me for weeks.

I spend the first few nights hidden in basements and attics of friends because everyone likes drafting off my rebellion. Once I sense that I've overstayed my welcome, I simply slip away.

After a week on the run, I sit behind a bakery on 9th East and 9th South and wonder what to do next. Last night I flattened myself into the shadows of a park, pulled my hoodie over my face, and tried to disappear. Homelessness is scarier at night.

Dad taught me how to sleep on ledges and under boulders and in snow caves, where we'd stack ropes and backpacks to insulate us from the cold earth. On those nights, we'd huddle and watch the stars as Dad told my brother and me the myths of constellations. He'd point and say, "That's Pegasus, Poseidon's stolen horse." Or "There is the great hunter Orion. Over there is Taurus the bull. Cory, that's your birth sign, which I think is bullshit." And "There's Ursa Minor, the little bear who's the son of Callisto. He's the most important because the tip of his tail is the North Star. If you can find Ursa Minor, you can orient yourself anywhere." In the park, I couldn't find the bear's tail and it was nothing like sleeping in the mountains. All I did was shiver and miss Dad and now I'm tired and my clothes are dirty and starting to smell sour. I never want to sleep in the park again. I miss Mom's peanut chicken.

A dawn shift worker slips out the side door of the bakery and lights a cigarette and I smell hot bread. He's wearing a dirty white apron over a tie-dyed shirt with the long sleeves pushed up to his elbows and fraying at the cuffs. He has cigarettes and I want one. "Can I give you a quarter for a smoke?" It's a generous bid considering I am down to seven dollars and a collection of pocket change that never adds up.

"I don't need a quarter." He hands me two cigarettes. I'm learning to play tough but he's kind and follows the gesture politely. "What's your name?"

"Thanks so much, man. Cory. What's yours?"

"Ryan. You're welcome."

Ryan is all punk rock with gauged earrings, tattoos, and short, messy blue hair with gray roots. He asks what year I am, and I tell him I would be a freshman. "Would be?" I tell him that my parents kicked me out because I'm perfecting a version of my story that generates sympathy—being kicked out makes my parents the villains and me the victim. I'm the heroic castaway, misunderstood and brilliant. I'm the wayward poet, tortured artist, and rebel. In this version of the story, I'm the brave anarchist betrayed by convention.

"Do you have a place to stay?" Ryan asks. I know I don't smell like I have a place to stay and look at my feet. "I get off at three.

Come back then . . . I live just around the corner. You can hang out there if you want." He hands me another cigarette before slipping back inside. I jog around the backside of the building and up the street and look for a quiet place to stare at a wall for the next five hours. Time always feels too slow on these days and Pink Floyd sings, "Ticking away the moments that make up a dull day / Fritter and waste the hours in an offhand way."

Just weeks before I was put in the hospital, I skipped class and ransacked my parents' liquor cabinet with a girl I'll call Kate. She was tall with short strawberry hair and didn't look like any of the fantasy girls in the magazines I kept under my mattress. But she was cool in an outcast kind of way and I liked her. Our faux nonconformity made us kindred.

We chose the sweetest alcohol we could find and poured shots, trying to calm our nerves because we came with a purpose. We weren't ready to have sex, but I don't imagine anyone ever is until they do. We weren't in love in the way we'd been told to be. We'd never held hands at a movie or swayed awkwardly at a dance. We were breaking all the romantic rules we'd been taught, chasing hormones and curiosity and an insatiable urge to discover something new about ourselves. More than anything, we wanted to be adults.

Our lips mashed together and I could taste the schnapps as I noticed all the wetness of teenage kisses. Within minutes, our bodies were sliding and pulsing and jerking with inelegant, unpracticed movements as we mimicked a version of what films and TV had taught us. Reality is much clumsier and messier. The smell of sex was visceral and pungent and new. But amidst all the awkwardness, I discovered a third place where my brain stops and I'm forced into presence, forgetting time aside from *now* in a blinding moment of connection to everything. I had nature and art. And now I had sex to stop my mind, however briefly.

At its worst, sex is forced, taken, violent, and a crime committed mostly by men. At its best, it's the sum of nature plus art. It's life's oldest and simplest math, an equation that has no real answer and makes sense only for a moment before collapsing back into the confusion of emotion.

That day it was very brief. Just as quickly as the noise of the world evaporated, it came rushing back and my thoughts were even louder than before. There was shock and shame and the recently intoxicating smell seemed gross. We cleaned ourselves and stripped the bed of bloody sheets and flipped the mattress and it felt like we were trying to hide it from ourselves as much as from anyone else. I wondered how something so natural could be so bewildering.

We walked back to the park in a haze and tried to make jokes the way lovers are supposed to. But we weren't lovers. We were just kids. And the thing that was supposed to make me feel grown up only made me feel like a child. We slid back into a circle of friends sitting in the park and told them we'd just gone for a walk. But they already seemed to know what happened and I wondered if they could smell us. Was I different from the person I'd been an hour before?

Time is the most-used word in the English language, and it's such a tricky thing. There are a finite number of times we get to do anything and after the first time it's a count. We only get to look at the sky so many times in a life. There are a finite number of rainstorms and seasons that we'll witness, and the number seems so big until it doesn't. We never know when will be the last time we taste something or see someone or do anything at all. And for all the money in the world, time is not for sale no matter what the doctors say when we beg for more of it toward the end, finally seeing that we forgot to count the raindrops.

After this first encounter I will chase sexuality and trade more time for it than anything else because for a moment *in time* I feel part of something so unifying that the separateness of my mind and body disappears. For a moment, sex fuses me back to myself and a body I only use but never inhabit. And because I'm briefly whole I can touch the world that I seem to have lost touch with.

In time it will drive the very dissociation I use it to overcome. The more of it I have, the more of it I'll need to feel anything, until I feel nothing at all but anger. I'll feel rage that I can't return to that instant when the world somehow made sense and all my many pieces found each other again. Briefly whole, I was allowed to feel loved, even if it was just our fingertips touching as I floated away from myself and everything else.

That day was the *first* time, and however confusing it felt, I knew that I could only do anything for the first time once. I tell you this now because you must know it before I walk into Ryan's house.

I follow him along the side of a duplex over uneven cement, past grooved brick and window frames with cracked paint. There's overgrowth that's swallowed a fence and makes it feel dark. A chain-link gate squeaks on its hinges and the lawn is weedy and dead and mostly dirt. I follow him inside through a flimsy screen door.

The living room is dim and I see that it needs to be vacuumed. I shower and use a towel that's still wet and smells like someone else. After putting on my dirty clothes, I sit on the couch while Ryan makes sandwiches, and this is what I know: He is nineteen. He works at a bakery. He lives in a house that has a dirty carpet. And he is gay. He tells me this and I wonder why because I don't really care but it seems important to him that I know.

I feel mostly "straight," but I've always had questions and been afraid of the answers. I have no romantic desire toward other boys, but I do have a fierce sexual fascination that confuses me. The available labels feel incomplete because there are really only three. You can be gay or straight. You can be a bisexual woman and that's considered sexy. But apparently being a bisexual man is just a layover on the way to being gay. I feel trapped by incomplete options, suspended between who I'm *supposed* to be and who I *know* I am. In time I'll learn new words like *sapiosexual* and *heteroflexible* and *fluid* and *queer,* which will tell me that many people feel like they have a limb hanging outside the hard confines of sexual binaries. Those new words are stories too, but they'll help fill the gray space between black and white.

I slouch on Ryan's crappy couch and am flooded by fear and excitement. I'm on the run with no place to go other than back to a cage. I have seven dollars and no home and any affection is better than none, and I think I might know why he needs to tell me he's gay.

After several days sleeping on the lumpy futon, there's a palpable tension between us.

"You don't have to sleep on the couch, you know." His voice is foreign, but it's all I have.

"So the floor is better?" I always turn to humor when I'm nervous. But he isn't talking about the floor and I know this and he knows that I know this.

"You could sleep with me." This isn't just his idea but mine too. I've hinted at it and teased it over the days because I want to know what it feels like. I want to know if maybe all my confusion can be solved by loving someone different.

He's close enough for me to notice the difference between the warmth of a woman and the heat of a man and I don't have time to respond before I feel his lips on mine and am trapped between my fear and curiosity and all the confusion of sex and love and power and submission and I kiss him back, uncertain if I'm doing it right. I've never kissed a boy and it feels misplaced. It doesn't quite fit and I don't like the way I can feel his stubble on my face and the way his breath tastes. For me, there's a sweetness to a girl's breath and the lips are softer and many things in this moment feel slightly off. But I don't resist. I kiss back harder, trying to make it fit.

He stands and holds my hand, which also feels strange, and leads me into his bedroom. It's dark and messy with a high, unmade twin bed shoved into a corner. I don't resist. I'm not interested in him, but his desire makes me feel wanted and safe because I don't know where I belong.

He's gentle but I fake pleasure as I feel discomfort and pain and wonder if Kate felt the same way. It's forced. Not by him but by me. I don't yet understand that consent is not singular, but an unfolding string of agreements made throughout any experience. I don't know that I can say *no* once I've said yes. He falls asleep with his arm slung across me, attempting to fill emotional distance with physical closeness the way mismatched lovers do. The cheap cotton sheets are sticky from sweat and I am too hot and too cold and I want the smell off me again. I stare at the ceiling and fight a nearly uncontrollable urge to run. I don't want any of this and it has nothing to do with him at all. And then I do it again the following night. And again. Because maybe if I do it enough it will feel right and I'll be home. In time, I'll learn that many people, especially women, feel this nearly constantly, trapped by the idea that they must or that they owe their sexuality in some misunderstood exchange. I'll feel this many times again, wanting only the closeness but not the touch.

I don't tell him that I'm leaving, but I write a note with an empty and emphatic "*Thank you!*" I don't want him to feel like he's done anything wrong or that my leaving is because of anything that's happened even though it is. I can't stand the house or the dim light or the carpet or the bed in the corner or the person

I am when I feel his hands on me, my face in a pillow. I feel hollow and know there's no light at the end of this tunnel. I can't look at myself for fear of what the mirror might reflect. Will I be there at all or am I a ghost? I have nowhere to go but I can't stay here and I slip out another door, invisible once more.

After a few more days killing time in the park or alleys and dodging truancy officers, someone calls my parents. I can't run anymore and, frankly, I'm terrible at being homeless. I admit defeat and am carted back in time to the decaying brick building to become a newcomer again without shoes or a belt.

The resident psychologist sits across from me as I lie back on his couch and cry tears of exhaustion. He has sharp features and a blue glass eye that sort of matches the other one and a new curly gray perm. I've never seen a man with a perm before. He's a good therapist and I usually like him. But not tonight. After two weeks on the run with no pills to swallow, all the chemicals had faded and I'd hardly slept a full night. He leans in as I tell him about Ryan. He tells me what happened was sexual assault, statutory rape in legalese. The law assumes coercion under the premise that a minor is legally incapable of offering consent. But I don't feel assaulted, and I don't like that he's trying to reframe my memory to match his interpretation. He asks me if I understand. In Freudian psychology, *nachträglicjkeit* is a term that describes deferred action, or "afterwardness." Basically, it explains trauma as a retroactive experience that comes in hindsight, consciously or unconsciously. In this view, trauma is in some ways more memory than experience itself. *Nachträglicjkeit* explains why someone might not register an event as traumatic until something triggers the memory and trauma response in them years later. Time allows us to understand an experience differently, recalling it through a new lens. It can take decades for people to finally understand what happened.

For now and forever in regard to Ryan, I don't feel like a victim even as I nod yes and cry. The therapist thinks I'm crying because I agree, but I'm crying because I'm rejecting my real feelings. I'm crying because I'm trying to make something work that doesn't, trying to bend to make myself fit somewhere, just as I had with Ryan.

I played an equal role in what happened and gave over to it freely. As much as I might not have necessarily *wanted* it, I was a willing participant. I don't believe that hindsight gets to sidestep culpability and the decisions I made. Eventually I'll fully grasp *nachträglicjkeit* and how complex trauma can be. Maybe Ryan knew better. But then again, maybe he was as confused as me. I'll always believe that nothing we did was "wrong," and that all the black and white that the therapist is clinging to is more about his misunderstanding than my own.

Sexuality is often fluid, especially when we're trying to discover ourselves as teenagers. As simple as the math is, sex is always complex and interactions are often complicated psychological affairs. I want to stand against the will of all the adults with so many opinions and certainties. I want to stand up for Ryan and the choices I made, however nuanced. But I don't. Instead, I'm taken on a field trip to identify his home and I want to vomit as I point from the car window, certain that I'm about to destroy a life in an irreversible way. I feel weak. The grown-ups want blood. I'm torn apart because some sinister piece of me likes this as much as I hate it. I like the attention and am willing to trade my truth for it. I'm betraying kindness.

The boat slams against the rocks. The mast is broken and the sails are torn. They want Ryan arrested and charged. As far as I know, that never happens. Still, Ryan, I'm sorry.

9

The second hand on my watch would twitch once, and a

year would pass, and then it would twitch again.

—Kurt Vonnegut, *Slaughterhouse-Five*

I f you know anything about my life (and that's a pretty big if), I imagine that some of you are wondering if I'm the same person who climbed mountains at all. I'm guessing that some are googling if there are two Cory Richardses and they've picked up the wrong memoir and are reading someone else's memories.

Mom taught me the most effective way to get anything done is to make a list, and I have a lot to do before I discover photography and rediscover the mountains and write this chapter. So I'll fast-forward. In film it's called a montage. And now a song sets in and scenes flash across the screen, condensing time and tying it all together with subtle symbolism. Some of these things you'll read more about later, but most of them you won't. They are as follows:

I'm fifteen the second time I run away from LifeLine. I use the head of a nail as a screwdriver to unlock a second-story window, escaping into the night with only a blanket and my boxer shorts. I'm captured the next day and dropped off at the squat red building on Foxboro Drive with no shoes and no small amount of shame.

The last time I abandon treatment, I don't run so much as walk out the front door because Mom and Dad concede defeat but tell me that I have no place to live. I sleep in more basements and attics next to things that are stacked and forgotten but not entirely thrown away and feel an affinity with the boxes that smell like dust. I sleep in the park and wonder if homeless people are closer to original humans, foraging in the forests that are buried under concrete and tennis courts and buildings.

Eventually family friends in Idaho take me in. They have three children around my age who do their best to accept me, but it's hard to assimilate. At night, I study for the General Educational Development (GED) test, which I joke stands for "Good Enough Diploma." After turning sixteen I pass the test and wonder if that's all I was really meant to learn in high school.

After eight months, I move back to Salt Lake as a sort of trial run at being home again and get a full-time job at a plant nursery that smells of fertilizer and potting soil. The soft background music is Paula Cole's "Where Have All the Cowboys Gone?" and the Wallflowers' "One Headlight" in a never-ending loop. I get fired after three months because I hate the music and stop showing up for work.

On weekends, I stand lookout while friends steal car stereos. I'm making poor life decisions and have started to steal things too: some money from Dad's private stash in his sock drawer, an unchained bike, a pager left on a table and ignored for one second too long. Eventually it all catches up when I'm arrested for shoplifting a pair of jeans.

It's all too much for Mom and Dad. This wasn't the agreement we made. So I sit outside the house and watch a locksmith change all the locks. With nowhere to go, I drive recklessly up a nearby canyon in a snowstorm until I smash through a guardrail and roll the car into a ravine. The engine has died, but the blinker is clicking and the windshield wipers are quietly thumping while my stolen radio continues to spin, but I can't hear the song.

Eventually I end up in Parowan, Utah, and try to get another

job, but no one is hiring. With nothing to do and no money, I slip
into a bottomless depression and return home as the prodigal son
after another flopped attempt at freedom. My brother is at the
house when I walk in, and it takes less than five minutes before
we're on the front lawn in a brawl. His arms are around my neck
as he tells me he's going to kill me. I drop to the ground and he
spits on me and drives away. I don't know where to put my emotions, so I kick out the windows in my car. The world is blurry
again, fogged up by thoughts that move too fast.

The following days, I'm back in the hospital where everything
is nailed to the floor and there's the familiar scent of burnt vacuum motors and antiseptic. The care team recommends a "fabulous program" for teens just like me! It's called LifeLine. They
obviously haven't bothered to read my file beyond checking
which prescriptions to fill. My parents see that despite all their
love, the care system itself is flawed and there might be no way to
"fix" me. I'm seventeen years old. The little boy with perfect
grades should be graduating next week and everyone wonders
where he's gone.

After a short negotiation with my parents, I move to Seattle
and live with Mom's youngest brother, Woody, and his wife,
Elise, who is a prettier version of Princess Diana. They have three
children, and now I'm a surrogate older brother and approach the
job with extreme care.

They're a devout family and I become deeply Christian after
going to church just once. I am "born again," both as a way to
belong to something and to rebel against Dad's stolid atheism.
He says, "Pray in one hand and shit in the other and tell me
which one fills up first." Amen. Like all my white-hot romances,
my love affair with Jesus won't last. In time I'll learn that faith is
often the messier of the two options. One you can hold. The
other can slip through your hands.

But for now, faith brings me peace and a sense of belonging.
In that security, I'm able to turn my gaze away from myself. I get

curious about the mountains again and climb Mt. Rainier with a friend and sleep on a high ridge above broken glaciers that fall away on both sides. The ice fades from black to brown to white as it crawls higher and higher into the sky. We listen to it groan and collapse in the darkness. I don't know that I've forgotten the sounds of high places until I hear them again. The next morning, we reach the summit just after dawn and the world is cotton-candy pink. The horizon fades from orange to powder blue to black and the brightest stars look like pinholes.

Having rediscovered a piece of myself that I didn't know I'd misplaced, I feel a sense of renewed passion and start climbing again. To support it all, I get three jobs and Woody takes half of every paycheck as "rent" and costs of living. But after eight months, he tells me he'll give all my money back if I choose an *experience* to spend it on. I choose to go to the Ruth Gorge in Alaska on a climbing trip with a group of Dad's old mountain partners. Adam, my best friend from childhood, joins as well. Before leaving, I ask Mom if I can borrow her 1984 Ricoh point-and-shoot camera. I'm eighteen and hungry for the life I seemed to have missed.

We fly into the Great Gorge in a bush plane and I feel small in a new way. Sharp granite faces rise from the glacier and I learn that, like me, mountains have many moods. They are mercurial and dangerous and beautiful. They are also uncaring, cold, and hostile. In these ways, I feel more mountain than human. The rock faces are streaked with ice and overhung by glaciers. We watch avalanches pour off and I hear the gravity of truly massive, high mountains. It is the sound of the earth spinning.

I take hundreds of pictures. Most are garbage. But something about this place and these motions agrees with me, and I discover a new place where my mind stops—another place where nature and art coalesce. I can freeze moments of meaning. It's an act of control in a life that has too often had none.

In base camp, I share a tent with Adam. He's quiet and

thoughtful with his words, and I think I can see a deep sadness in his eyes but I don't know what I'm looking at. He's also playful and loves to fart and push the smell my way. Fifteen years from now, Mom will cry on the phone and tell me Adam has hung himself and I'll finally recognize the pain that existed in the tent. I'll dig for the pictures I took of him, but they'll be lost and I'll understand just how important a photo can be.

At Woody's urging, I decide to go back to school and tour a Christian college in Reading, California, where I'll study to become a youth pastor so I can share my troubled past alongside my infallible faith in Jesus. But there are cracks in my faith, and the fractures widen when a pastor suggests that the world is six thousand years old, carbon dating is false, and dinosaur bones were put in the ground by a loving God who will test our faith and cast us into eternal damnation if we don't pass the fossil record quiz. I do not become a youth pastor.

Instead, I drive to Montana and start school at Rocky Mountain College and study English. In my War Literature class, I read Hemingway and Vonnegut and Heller and O'Brien, and Joseph Conrad says, "The horror. The horror." I wonder how a loving God can permit so much pain if we are created in his image.

Over spring break, I drive to Zion National Park alone, intent on soloing the sheer sandstone walls. I meet John in a parking lot on the first morning. He looks like he's part Viking, part Greek God and talks loudly and tells filthy jokes. I abandon my solo aspirations five minutes after meeting him. Together, we spend the week climbing varnished Navajo Sandstone sweating, swearing, and laughing and I like the small scabs on my hands and the way they bleed. We sleep 1,500 feet above the canyon floor in a hanging cot called a portaledge and wax philosophical, which is an easy thing to do when your legs are dangling into a void. We smoke hand-rolled cigarettes and shiver through desert nights, and I notice that climbing has a way of making life feel lighter by amplifying the risks of gravity. For the first time I can remember, I am truly at peace. I'm also looking for brothers, and I learn that the risk of climbing forms deep bonds exceptionally quickly.

Back in Montana, I manage to hold a job at a gear store, and during the summer between my freshman and sophomore years, John, Adam, and I go to Alaska to climb Denali. I feel small on the way up and enormous on the way down. I'm nineteen years old.

Halfway up the mountain, we're camped on a small glacial plateau. On a rest day, I wander around the expanse and make a photograph of ski tracks that lead toward an edge that falls away, revealing the enormousness of the Alaska Range in the distance. The weight of the skier compacted the snow as the friction of the ski turned the track to ice. When the wind blew away the loose snow around the tracks, they were left raised above the surrounding surface. I watch the scene in silence and like the idea of taking pictures of people that have no people in them. I'm discovering the nuance of photography and how to say more by showing less.

Two weeks after returning home from Alaska, John and I board another plane for Peru, and I learn that every place has a smell. Lima smells like concrete, steel, spice, and guinea pig cooked on the street, all mixed with thick, salty air that blows off the sea. We take an overnight bus to Huaraz and spend four weeks in the Cordillera Blanca, and I take more pictures. The fractured pieces of me seem to be fusing back together.

I'm still mercurial, but I haven't been depressed or hypomanic for years. They call this remission, and it's common after a first major episode of bipolar. It's also when someone rejects their diagnosis and stops taking their medication because obviously the doctors were wrong and it was just a moment and now my brain is better and Mom asks, "Are you still taking your medications?" I am, but I hate the pills because they remind me of the past.

I buy a micro-tip pen and make a note on every slide of where each photograph was taken and draw a copyright symbol next to my name in meticulous block letters. I learn what a masthead is and where to find it in magazines and catalogs that accept free-lance submissions. Sliding the images of my three "expeditions" into a FedEx envelope, I'm filled with confidence. I mail it to the Patagonia photo department, certain that it will be returned with a check for untold thousands because I'm the undiscovered talent of my generation.

While I wait for my check, I read the Gospel of Matthew, where Jesus says, "Some [seed] fell on rocky places, where it did not have much soil. It sprang up quickly, because the soil was shallow. But when the sun came up, the plants were scorched, and they withered because they had no root." After three tumul-tuous years with Jesus, I let go of my faith and wander into a new future, less bound by guilt and shame.

When the slides are returned three months later, there's no check. Instead, I pull out a thin piece of paper with a note in typewriter font (as all letters concerning art should be). It reads:

Dear Cory,

Thank you so much for your submission to the Patagonia Photo Dept. After careful consider-ation, we've determined that we don't have a place for any of your images at this time. You have some great work here and I encourage you to keep submitting.

Sincerely,

Jane Sievert

P.S. I think you can turn off the date and time-stamp feature of your camera.

In the corner of every slide is a bright orange time and date burned into the film, and I'm learning how much I don't know about photography and cameras and pictures. All artists are rejected before they're embraced, I think. But more important, the letter is proof that I exist in a new, more hopeful world.

The montage ends now. I'm twenty years old.

10

They say seeing is believing, but the opposite is true.

Believing is seeing.

—ERROL MORRIS

The next twenty-two years of my life begin in a cave in Salzburg, Austria. After Denali and Peru, my wanderlust piqued and I impulsively applied to study abroad. Either by clerical error or a stroke of luck, I was accepted into the program, and here I am.

The old city wraps around the Mönchsberg, the Monk's Mountain, which is named after the Benedictine monks of St. Peter's Abbey, founded in A.D. 696. It's a steep mound of crushed river stone with a white medieval fortress on top. The city is magical and many great minds were born here. Christian Doppler observed the frequency of waves, Hans Makart revolutionized painting, and Mozart was born in a tall yellow house that I'm sure was a different color at the time. Most days, the city has the rich organic smell of manure and I wonder where it comes from.

In 1558, a townhouse was built using the cliff of the Mönchsberg as the back wall. On the third floor is a white room with a door that leads to a small cave that is full of humid musk. The organic scent of stone mixes with a hint of chemicals that I learn to call developer and fixer. It's the first darkroom I've ever been in, and it glows red, is always warm, and is neatly packed with enlargers and developing stations. This is the room that changes the direction of everything.

Andrew Phelps is my photography teacher for the semester and I like him immediately. He's "tall, dark, and handsome," a bit lanky, and I notice his cheekbones. He has short messy hair that is fine but not thinning, and his eyes are framed by thin lines as if he's been squinting his whole life, looking for things that no one else sees.

Andrew is a fine-art photographer whose images are complex and simple at the same time, mysterious because they seem to be at battle with themselves. They reflect a deep understanding of photographic principle and theory, which I know nothing about. For me, photography is literal and impulsive, like I'm trying to catch moments falling past me. But his are deliberate, crafted, and made, not taken. They're responses to the world, not reactions to it.

I show him my binder of pictures that jump and have no order and no consistent style. I'm all eyes and no voice and the images seem as scattered as my brain. One of the first things he tells me is that sometimes the best way to find a voice is to shut up, suggesting that I let the world talk for a moment instead of thrusting myself upon it.

At the end of my first semester he gives me two rolls of film. My assignment is to walk the trails of the Mönchsberg in silence like a Benedictine friar and make something beautiful out of a pile of sticks or a wall or a hamburger wrapper. He's teaching me not to rely on the fantastic but rather to develop the skill of seeing magic in the mundane because that is where most of life happens. Photography is alchemy, he says. It's not simply pressing a button but choosing where to point the camera with studied anticipation. It's the serendipity of moment and light and there are no mistakes, just lessons.

After two weeks I pin my collection of pictures to the wall and it looks like I've gone around photographing people's gardening piles. They're muted and dull and someone in the class says, "Soooo . . . you just took pictures of sticks?" I'm angry because these sticks took a lot of effort. I'm impatient but also know that mastery takes more than just a semester abroad. I want to be great *now*, but Andrew is patient.

It's summer between semesters and I'm living in a tent behind a hedonistic hostel in Interlaken, Switzerland, which is appropriately called the Funny Farm. Unlike the hospitals of my past, the hostel is a joyful sort of "crazy," but the screams sound the same. I flip burgers and roll joints for the pretty American girls I try to sleep with.

One gives me crabs and I find myself in a pharmacy pantomiming my discomfort to a pharmacist by scratching wildly at my groin because I don't know the German word for crabs (it's *krebs*). The Lonely Planet phrasebook does not include "I have crabs" or "My crotch has fire ants" or "I'm a dirty little slut, please help." The people in line behind me giggle as the pharmacist hands me shampoo and a tiny comb and carefully explains exactly how to use it to get rid of my *krebs*.

I clean the rat's nests of hair clogging the shower drains and pick up used condoms and mop the vomit of a frat boy who drank too much. I wash the sheets of a drunk kid from Philly who pissed the bed and clean the deep fryer and mop the grease from the kitchen floor. I save all the money and rent a broom-closet apartment in Chamonix, France, where I devote myself to climbing and photography for the remainder of the summer.

The north face of the Aiguille du Midi falls away into darkness under my feet. Chamonix twinkles 4,000 feet below us and I think of Dad and the first time I bivouacked. *Bivouac* is a French word for "sleep here without a tent, dumdum." Dad taught my brother and me how to make a lumpy mattress from ropes and packs and climbing gear and that your hips will always hurt and that bivouac doesn't always mean "sleep." That night with Dad and my brother we slept under a boulder in the Wind River Range, which had the added benefit of being sheltered from the wind. Tonight I'm with Stian Hagen and Jamie Straichan and it's warm and breathless.

A serac cracks and falls, thundering down the face to our left, and the last bits of ice tinkle in the quiet that follows. Tonight there is joy in suffering because I'm not suffering too much. I'm learning how little I need to be safe in the mountains, though not always comfortable.

In big mountains and on serious climbs, slow is dangerous and learning what to bring and what to leave is its own special art. The more you bring the slower you climb, which means more time under melting ice cliffs and falling rocks. Longer days mean a deeper fatigue, which is harder to recover from during uncomfortable nights when sleep is sparse. Slow means exposure to heavy avalanches that are thicker than concrete and literally pull your body apart as you suffocate. Over a career, slow increases your chances of *décès,* which is French for "dirt nap," which is climber slang for dying. The cost of safety in the mountains is often paid in discomfort and hunger while still having enough energy to keep going. But if you overestimate your tolerance for suffering, there is the risk of being too exposed and too cold and being forced down before you tip over the edge. Climbing is an art of balance.

The morning is cold and crisp as Stian hangs all the dangly metal bits of gear from his harness and starts to climb. The granite is cold, and my fingers are dry and skinny from dehydration. We climb 1,000 feet of easy terrain until the stone becomes snow just as the sun peaks. The valley is blue and sleeping as Stian follows me up a narrow rib of ice. Behind him, a jagged tooth of sunny rock breaks the shadows below. I point my camera and take eight pictures. Picture four will be my first published image.

Photography is an art of hundredths and thousandths of seconds, which makes for slim odds at perfection. The moment of any image is preceded by an infinite number of events that coalesce in a single instant, and it evaporates just as quickly as it appears. It's vanishingly rare to know that you've made a near-perfect picture. After twenty years I'll be able to count on two hands the number of times that I *knew* it was happening, that I *felt* it. All the rest will be luck and knowing where to look with a sort of refined anticipation. But this morning is the first time I *feel* a picture and know it's special.

Some drugs you only need to do once to fall into a hopeless addiction because the potency of the rush is so complete. It's as if you've discovered a piece of yourself that you didn't know existed and now you're somehow incomplete without it. You'll kill yourself to feel alive and connected in the same way and I hear myself reciting the first step of recovery: *I admit that I am powerless, and my life has become unmanageable.* I'm powerless in the face of this moment and I think, "Fuck manageable . . . I'd die for this."

It's the end of my second semester in Salzburg and I've taken many pictures while nearly failing every other class because I only care about one thing. I'm standing in Andrew's studio looking at an old piece of paper tacked to the wall. Block letters in faded permanent marker say simply, *PROCEED AND BE BOLD.*

"What's this about?" I ask. Andrew is shuffling through prints behind me and says, "This path isn't easy and you're definitely not

gonna get rich. But if you want my opinion, you should take it."
It's all the encouragement I need. Neither of us knows the gravity of his words.

The days are short and gray and wet without snow or rain. Andrew drives me to the train station as triangles of ice float in the Salzach River like bumper cars. We're talking about nothing and pointing to things that no one else might see.

"Look at the shape that building makes."

"It's weird that days can be black and white like this."

"Aside from the stoplights."

He's squinting through the windshield looking for a turn. "You have all the pieces to be very good at this," he says over the heater. "But if I can give you just one piece of advice? Never let photography become who you are. It can't be that. It's just something you do." I wonder if he is talking to himself as much as me and I don't understand at all.

I step out of the car into the familiar scent of manure that always comes before the snow. "I wish there was a way to photograph the smell of cow shit . . ."

Andrew laughs. "Proceed and be bold."

11

That's how the madness of the world tries to colonize

you: from the outside in, forcing you to live in its reality.

—JEFF VANDERMEER

've always had nightmares. In one I'm running from something that has no form. It's dark and nameless, but my legs can't move fast enough, as if I am sprinting in a swimming pool and going nowhere. The shape never catches me but is always over my shoulder. This is the nightmare I have most.

In another my teeth are falling out and I can feel the shards in my mouth like sharp pebbles and sand that crunches. I try to spit them out but more teeth fall away until my jaw detaches and I'm holding it in my hand. I struggle to put it back on but instead extract a piece of my spine. The bones are soft, as if they've been boiled, and fall apart in my hands in mush.

In the third I fall from a cliff. This one I've learned to control. I can slow my plunge and glide until I land. The impact is always hard, but I'm unhurt. I never fly, but I never die either.

But now I'm having a new nightmare of oversized American flags above enormous, half-full parking lots. Loose snow is slithering its way across icy asphalt like the ghosts of snakes. There are big-box stores like Best Buy and Target and chain restaurants like Fuddruckers and Golden Corral where old people go to get the early bird special for $5 and eat mashed potatoes and chicken-fried steak and creamed corn. There's a big billboard that says *Meth: Not Even Once* under a picture of a girl with unwashed hair and dark eyes. She has open sores and her teeth are falling out. I run my tongue over mine to make sure they're still there and that I'm not going to lose my spine. Another billboard says *JesUSAves—John 14:6* and I wonder how faith can be so concrete and porous all at once. The big white landscape is dotted by dead cottonwood trees that look like ghosts behind gusts of loose snow. My heat doesn't work and I'm shivering and the CD is skipping but I can't take my hands off the wheel because the tires are slipping. This dream is about home and history. I'm being haunted and told it is time to move on.

When I come home from Europe, I don't go back to Montana but drive to Seattle and rent a 375-square-foot apartment. It's a "studio" when I'm an artist and a "cell" when I crash back into depression, which has returned in short bursts. It lasts for a week. Sometimes two. I never see it coming and only know I'm in it once I start trying to crawl my way out.

Every day I walk fifteen minutes to the Art Institute of Seattle, where I've enrolled in the photography program. At night, I work at a climbing gym that smells of chalk and sweat, where I build a small community of friends that will guide my early adventure career. Steve Swenson. Jesse Huey. Shane Chelone. Scott Zaleski. Kevin Battey. I'm usually late to work and am let go after a year, which is fine with me because I've started working as a photo assistant for Barb Penoyar, who laughs as loudly as she swears. When I meet her, I'm studying photography from the Great Depression and she reminds me of a Dorothea Lange portrait because she's all grit and sturdy beauty and sadness and hope expressed as one. She's tempestuous like me and I know that her long silences do not come from inner peace. She drinks until her head hurts and we share a silent language of pain and creativity that connects us beyond student and teacher. I fear and adore her.

In exchange for mopping and painting the floors, and running countless errands to the film lab, she gives me a key to the studio, where I can make my own pictures and learn the technical skills of lighting. I stay late and come early and when I'm not working for her I sit on the freshly painted floor and devour photography: Jodi Cobb. Alex Webb. William Allard. Sebastião Salgado. Avedon. Newton. Lindbergh. Ritts. Leibovitz. Benson. These are the names I learn first, unaware of how big the world of photography is. These photographers are masters, but they can overshadow an entire ocean of talent. In time, I'll learn that fame isn't necessarily synonymous with great art.

I buy *Climbing* magazine and *National Geographic* and look at who shot what and try to understand why some rules are broken and others are followed and why some blurry images with terrible light and no composition are the best. I want to know why some photos rise above the swill of mediocrity and how they do it. It's my own theory, but I learn that there are really only four kinds of pictures in the world.

There are many good pictures, and they combine light and composition with subject and environment. A bad photographer can be taught to make good pictures and might even become a decent photographer.

There are far fewer great pictures because they're much harder to make. The compositions are more articulate and rely on anticipation and tension and mood. They follow all the rules but in a different way. A naturally good photographer can evolve and make great pictures, but it's rare because the skills aren't taught but discovered through repetition and curiosity. These pictures are driven by a deeper understanding of concept and theory.

Then there are *transcendent* images, which are the rarest of all. Sometimes they have shitty light and no concept. They can be ill-composed and a big blurry mess. A naked child runs with outstretched arms, screaming from the burn of napalm. Nick Ut. A monk sitting in lotus, dead calm and engulfed in flames. Quang Duc. A man fires a pistol into the head of another on the street in Saigon. Eddie Adams. A man jumps a puddle and hovers for a moment. Henri Cartier-Bresson.

Ironically, *anyone* can make a transcendent picture because they don't trade on technicality. They're based on moment and emotion and serendipity and luck. Being skilled or talented just increases the chances of getting one because you're looking and more often in the right place at the right time to observe the fantastic and heartbreaking. I discover this on Barb's white floor and photography begins to make sense in a new way. I wonder if pictures of climbing and exploration can ever be transcendent. Maybe.

The fourth kind of image is the most common of all. Bad pictures. I will take many of these.

The two most common words that will be used to describe my photography are *emotional* and *raw*. I'll make many good pictures and a handful of great ones. I'll never make a transcendent picture. But there will be one powerful enough to exalt and destroy me.

Barb introduces me to another photographer named Bill Cannon. He has short salt-and-pepper hair and perfect wrinkles around bright blue eyes that always look boyish. Bill has no time for bullshit and fires me countless times only to rehire me because for all his hardness he's one of the most patient people I'll ever know. But now he's usually whisper-yelling at me and saying, "Your job is not to fuck models and when you're trying, they're talking, and you're fucking up my film. This is a job, not a bar. Get your shit together!" I apologize but keep flirting anyway.

Bill's first assistant is named Mark Stone and is the buffer between us, keeping me in line while keeping Bill calm and reminding him that if he fires me he's just going to hire me again anyway. We're in San Diego and Miami and Charleston. I'm packing the cameras and getting on a flight and showing up early and going home late, learning never to be the one who keeps the production waiting. I learn to shut up and do my job. We're in the Florida Keys and Santa Barbara and New York. Bill fires me. Bill hires me. Mark laughs while I absorb lighting and framing and everything else that makes a photograph work. Mark will eventually become my assistant, which is a terrible word for what he really is, which is co-author, co-conspirator, creative partner, dear friend, therapist, and, above all, brother.

When insomnia grabs hold of me, I wander out into the drizzly underworld of downtown Seattle. Neatly stacked islands of light stretch down the long streets and I hear voices that echo and bottles that tinkle in the shadows. Lack of sleep never occurs to me as an indication that I might be cycling up or down. I just have more energy or am too tired to rest. So I sleuth the shadows, photographing the schizophrenic and the addict and the prostitute and empty streets, playing a game of freeze tag with hungry ghosts and future versions of myself. There is nothing new or original in my photographs and I'm frustrated to know it. This work has been done a million times before. For me, it's a sort of exploitative study. I wonder if it will ever be me screaming at things that no one else sees. The doctors warned me of this. Maybe if I give my own darkness a voice, my teeth will stop falling out and I won't keep slow-running and falling off cliffs. As much as I'm making pictures of what I'm seeing, I'm also photographing the things I fear in myself.

When the sun comes out, I go climbing.

"Watch me!" I yell down to Jesse. It's code for "I'm scared and I'm probably going to fall." He yells up from 100 feet below, "I've got you," and I lunge for a tiny granite ledge. My hands and feet leave the rock and for a moment, no piece of me is connected. When my fingers come back to the stone, they instantly slip off and I fall. I hang on the end of the rope, which always seems too thin to hold me, and spin in space, looking up at the moves I can't quite do. These days, climbing is an undertaking of joy and struggle and suffering and a conduit for all of life boiled down to a singular act. It's a title bout with gravity that captures all emotions and forces them on display.

Climbing is an act of overcoming through reduction and refinement and occasionally brute force. Try too hard here and you'll have none left. Don't try hard enough and you'll fall. At the upper edge of anyone's ability, placing a hand or foot a millimeter differently in any direction is often the deciding blow.

I still don't feel like I fit anywhere, but I can ignore that here. My relentless drive toward the extreme is both a reflection of my mind and a way to reconnect with a body that I have learned to dissociate from. The pictures are a way to try to understand emotion by freezing it. They're a way to feel and my best attempt to unify all the pieces of me that seem to be otherwise disconnected.

"You got this!" Jesse calls up. I reluctantly paw for the rock, lock my fingers onto a tiny ledge, and pull.

I have a sense that the further I'm willing to go and the more I'm willing to risk, the less likely I am to sleep in the alleys and scream at trees. The decision to pursue my own edges by pushing the limits of my safety is not a conscious one and I don't know when I make it. It will not just be climbing. It will be traversing ice caps and rivers in Africa and forgotten seas and I'll lose sight of land and the world altogether. It will nearly kill me many times. This decision will precipitate heartbreak and selfishness and elation and success and shocking moments of joy and campfires and long nights of looking at nothing. The highs will be dizzying and the lows will be suicidal at times. I'll collect many brothers and sisters and will hurt many friends when I withdraw. They'll feel used. Some will forgive me, and others won't, and many will lose faith in my friendship because I'm as unreliable as my moods. I'll learn that there is little room for others when we're consumed by ourselves.

Many friends will die and I'll wish that I'd been better to them. At times it will seem senseless. But I'll ignore the warning of mortality. I'll be criticized by many and adored by others. I won't be the best and some people will hate me and think my success is undeserved. A piece of me will agree while another laps up the adoration of everyone who offers it. I'll drink and fuck in celebration. I'll do the same to escape the isolation of the choice I'm about to make.

It's irrational but I can see no other solution even though I can't see now what I'm doing at all. I'm not only trying to unify myself but also to put as much distance between me and an inevitable madness clipping at my heels. I'm always scared but the fear also drives me, feeding the pieces of my brain that thrive in chaos. I won't understand any of it until I break on a mountain nineteen years from now. The decision is an outright and unbridled expression of my unquiet mind. I'm choosing a life of polarity. In order to escape madness, I will live madly. I will risk my life in order to save it.

I board a flight for Australia and the Coral Sea.

II

12

Why is a raven like a writing desk?

—The Mad Hatter

've never sat in a sea kayak, but it's only a thousand miles. Averaging twenty-four miles a day, that's 41 days. Which is 984 hours. Which is 59,040 minutes. Which is 3,542,400 seconds. I'm twenty-three and my cracked watch is slowly filling with saltwater, corroding and rusting. I like the way it looks as I float on an open sea and wonder again about time.

For indigenous Australians, the past and present are apprehended in a cyclical order of creation and formlessness that is both ancient and now. Ancestorial histories are lived, daily expressions of morality and rules for life and interactions with the natural world. In English, it's called the Dreaming, and as much as it's a creation story, it is an all-embracing concept that is not fixed in time. Rather, it *is* time and everything in it all at once. The Dreamtime happens in the Everywhen. The Dreamtime *is* the Everywhen.

As I consider the formless nature of time, I'm learning that a boat moves in six ways: heave, sway, surge, pitch, roll, and yaw. We are six people in six kayaks. Six dots of color. We have six stories. Six ways of saying good morning and six definitions of love. Six ways of saying "I hate this." Six versions of risk and six senses. Six ideas of time and everything in it. We are on one long journey, paddling 1,000 miles of northern Queensland's forgotten coast from Cairns to the tip of the continent and into the Torres Strait.

I think of the number six as I learn that the trough between ocean waves is a dismal place. Everything disappears as it's swallowed by walls of water. For a moment you are utterly alone. Wind hits the top of the swells and rains down on me and I know if I allow too many waves to rise and fall, I will lose sight of my partners altogether. This terrifies me because there are monsters in the water below.

Two scare me the most. Saltwater crocodiles love this sea and grow as long as 20 feet, and we call them "salties." Box jellyfish breed here too and have long tentacles and toxic venom so powerful it's said to produce the deepest pain humans know and stings are often fatal. Whenever I'm in the trough between waves, both creatures feel closer, hidden just out of sight.

The peak of a wave is a calming albeit momentary relief from the trough and I can see everything for one brilliant instant. But the view of everything reveals nothing but sea and I long for the trough again. The trough feels small by comparison. The trough is safe because the open sea is too big. No mountain has made me feel insignificant in the way the ocean does. No snow has made my eyes burn this much. The only comfort is the red needle of a compass pointing north and knowing that somewhere to my left there is land.

The surface area of the Coral Sea off the eastern coast of Australia is 1,850,000 square miles, which is a lot of space to stare at from the peak of a wave. The total surface area of a sea kayak is a matter of several square feet, and I sit a few inches above the water, locked in a cramped cockpit that is always wet. If it's ever dry, my legs rub against grains of sand that never wash out and my crotch sweats so much that I hold my breath every time I open the spray skirt to avoid the blast of stagnant humid air that smells of rubber and mildew and vinegar.

Every day is the same. After a few hours, my ass and hips are in excruciating pain because it doesn't matter how molded the seat is or how soft the hip pads are. If I'd known the pain I'd be in and if I'd known the magnitude and audacity of this undertaking and if I'd known how scared I'd be, I never would have agreed to this.

When saltwater seeps into scrapes, nicks, bug bites, and open sores, the edges of the wounds rise in a soft white perimeter of flesh that never dries. After a week calluses form on the protruding bones of my pelvis. After two weeks I hardly feel any sensation at all because after enough troughs and peaks, I no longer notice any of it. The sum of my existence is just an ache behind my shoulder blades, a dull hum in my neck, and a sinewy sensation that runs from my armpits to my waist and I can't tell where my body stops and my kayak starts.

At times I'm bored of awe and hardly see the beauty at all. At other moments I'm awed at the depth of my boredom. Eventually I'm no longer scared of the 20-foot saltwater crocodiles when they surface and dive in front of my bow. When I land on the beach, I look for the tracks of their enormous tails sliding in and out of the surf. These tracks are known as "slides"; if they're there I ignore them, and I wonder if being unafraid of a prehistoric killing machine has nothing to do with courage but is its own special kind of stupid.

I notice small rings of salt forming around the buttons and dials on my cameras. Saltwater has now filled my watch and trapped a piece of the sea forever. Film canisters show signs of rust and corrosion and I shoot more images than I've ever taken but have no idea if they're any good as I tuck the rolls into a waterproof bag.

We plan to refill our dwindling water supply at a spring along a hopelessly isolated piece of coast because it's the only water for miles and we have none left. But the spring is dry. The Millennium Drought of the 2000s has just been declared the worst in Australia's recorded history.

The next morning, I wake with my five companions and wander into the hot, scratchy forest, known to Australians as the "bush." Dry leaves crunch under my feet as I bushwhack through an unending maze of spiderwebs and follow choked drainages where water runs in the rainy season. But there isn't a rainy season this year. Eventually we find a tiny puddle of mud with some wet leaves that smell of decay and dig a hole until dirty, reddish iron-filled water fills the depression. We alternate carrying twenty-liter jugs back to camp, watching for snakes as we sweat through our clothes. When we're back on the beach, we discover that all our cheese has been eaten by dingoes and I remember a jovial Australian calling Foster's Lager "dingo piss." Right now I'd cut off a pinky to drink some dingo piss.

One night we sleep on Lizard Island, where there is a fancy hotel. Before Europeans and five-star resorts, the Dingaal people called the island Dyiigurra. To them, it was a sacred place for the initiation of boys into manhood. For them, it was created during the Dreamtime, the Everywhen, when magic existed and creation was unfolding, as it is now too. They saw it as the body of a stingray. On August 12, 1770, Captain Cook named it Lizard Island when he climbed to its peak to chart a course through the reef and something ancient became something new and something eternal was now finite because one thing becomes another while it remains unchanged. That is how time works in the Everywhen.

Some days the water is clear and shallow and I glide over miles of bright corals, turtles, sharks, and stingrays. Some nights I sleep under the stars on forgotten islands of the Great Barrier Reef. There are no lights and I imagine what it must have been like a thousand years ago but realize how stupid the question is because it was just like this.

One afternoon, I sit on the beach and watch an endangered hawksbill turtle flip her way slowly from the surf. I don't move and she doesn't care, passing close enough for me to touch her shell, but I keep my hands to myself. She pushes and pulls and shoves her way across the beach, digs a hole, buries her eggs, and appears to weep as excess salt is expelled through her eyes. She was born nearby and has been swimming in large circles, pushed by currents and following invisible magnetic fields, returning over and over to this beach for longer than I've been alive. It's dark when she crawls back into the sea with sand covering her eyeballs and I imagine the relief she feels as the grit is washed away. I wonder how many of the eggs will survive.

Some days I lose control of my boat and the bow moves in every direction and I feel frenzied and confused until I discover that one of my teammates has flipped my rudder out of the water as a joke. Sometimes it's funny. Sometimes I want to rip the hands off whoever did it.

In the same way, some days I lose control of my mind. Like my boat, it moves in every direction, and I feel out of control and panic as the enormousness of the sea traps me. There's nowhere to be and everywhere to go and it's claustrophobic because it's so big and open, and I wonder who flipped up the rudder of my brain because it's not funny. I want to rip my own hands off. So every morning and night I take the pills that are supposed to keep me sane but wonder if they're working because all of this is insane.

I am a thousand years ago as I watch a plane fly overhead.

Two of my teammates move their tents away from the rest so they can have loud, sweaty sex and I'm mad when I hear them but am really just jealous. I'll grow to despise one teammate. I'll grow closer to others. One I never really know at all.

One night I wander away from the team because I need to be

alone and stand on a rocky point in bare feet and fish with a hand line. I swing the lure like a lasso until it gets momentum and then let it fly into the waves where the water is deep and clear and I watch the metal sparkle as it sinks. I reel in giant trevally (although the ones I catch aren't actually giant) and walk back to camp, triumphant. Food is simple but simple things are big when the goal is survival. We fillet the fish without cooking it and eat sashimi, parasites and all.

Another evening I wade into the shallow surf of a nameless island and catch a small barracuda. Another day I use a sling spear to kill reef sharks because we've run out of food, and we cook shark steaks on an open fire. One day we buy two kilos of shrimp from a trawler and have a feast on the beach, where we discover that coconuts have a soft spot that can be punctured with a pocketknife. We drink the water inside and mix it with rum and I'm Captain Jack Sparrow seven years before Johnny Depp and say, "But why is the rum gone?"

Every night we have a fire and stare at it until it glows dark red. We push our toes into the warm sand and we call this "watching bush TV." I look at my watch but there is no point because hours don't matter here.

After three weeks we pull our boats into a mangrove forest near Lockhart River and wander through the mud, watching for sleeping crocodiles until we find a shack where a hermit lives. He has a long silver beard and his mustache is stained from smoking hand-rolled cigarettes. I ask for one and smoke with him in silence because even though we both know English we can't communicate. We're from the same world but different times. The hermit's feet are swollen purple balloons at the bottom of two leather twigs interrupted by bulbous, arthritic knees with skin stretched so tight it shines. He shows us a shotgun, which is not a threat but a way to talk.

A man in a pickup truck collects a few of us and we drive into Lockhart River, population 497, for a resupply. Dave and I go to the bar because all I've been thinking about is beer. *Bar* is a generous description; it's a cement-block structure with cash windows that are covered by thick steel bars. Throngs of dark faces wander in all at once as if a whistle has blown somewhere in the bush. These are the faces of Native Australians, the faces of the Everywhen.

There is joy here and someone says, "Where ya from, mate?"

"America."

"What the fuck ya doin' here?"

"We're kayaking from Cairns to the tip."

"Ya crazy cunt. I don't believe ya!" We laugh.

We are the only white faces and I feel that we aren't entirely welcome even though no one asks us to leave. We're not to be trusted. Why would we be? We'll leave in kayaks tomorrow and almost everyone else will never leave at all.

For now, all I understand is that I'm afraid of the poverty and distrustful eyes that don't hate me but seem to resent the world I come from. This is the first, blistering moment of waking up to an ugly truth. I'll have this same feeling many more times all over the world, every face with a different story. Each with the same story. It's not a white man's tragic interpretation. It's a white man's footprint, which seems to be on someone's head.

I think of *Robinson Crusoe,* where Daniel Defoe wrote, "Thus we never see the true state of our condition till it is illustrated to us by its contraries, nor know how to value what we enjoy, but by the want of it." It's interesting that a book born of racism could miss the potency of its own words. I feel some sort of timeless guilt for which I'm not responsible but am part of nonetheless. We leave the following day with fresh supplies, and I'm ashamed of my relief. That is my ugly gift and I hate how grateful I am.

After forty-one days the bow of my kayak slides onto the beach just off Douglas Street on Thursday Island in the Torres

Strait and I weep because this has been the hardest thing I've ever done. I feel a million miles away from everyone because I know that life as a castaway is about to dissolve and I'll fly back into a world where everything is too fast and the only way to make it slow down is to match its pace.

I book a one-way flight back to Cairns while the rest of the team tries to paddle to Papua New Guinea. I tell them it's about schedule, but I'm lying. I'm scared. I'm scared of the coming depression. The trough of a wave is always equal to its peak. I'm scared of continuing because I'm too tired, too extended, too exposed, and too unmoored. Besides, my pills are almost gone. I want the safety of home but fear the depression it signals even though I will have plenty of pills there.

The air-conditioned plane flies south over the coast and I wonder who is looking up at me from a thousand years ago. It takes an hour to reverse the effort of 1,000 miles of fishing with hand lines and scavenging for food. A pretty flight attendant pours water in a thin plastic cup and I'm surprised to notice it's not iron-laden and red. I wonder if the short flight is erasing everything that I thought just happened, if I have gone back in time, or if it has been standing still.

When I get home, I deposit two dry bags that smell like cheese at the photo lab. The corroded film canisters inside are scratched and sandy. I look at thousands of pictures from the trip and try to sell them to magazines and kayak companies and apparel brands and two decades will pass without selling a single one or seeing anything in print.

My best friends throw a small party and draw pictures of penises on white T-shirts because they call me Dick Richards or Dick Dick. I laugh and feel loved and missed. I get drunk every night for the next week and try to feel like I'm "home."

I try to tell them about Australia and the Coral Sea and the indigenous concept of the Everywhen, but the conversation ends after five minutes because no one can understand any of it and I can't either and as much as I hated it at times, I realize that all I really want is to be back on a deserted coast, eating raw fish.

I sleep on the floor and stare at the ceiling and try to see through it. I know that I've just gone as far beyond the edge of comfort as I ever have and see that the edges are fast becoming the only place I feel comfortable at all. I'm always two versions of myself and I wake up in my bed confused.

My watch rusts airtight and traps a piece of the Coral Sea inside and it tells me it's three in the afternoon. I'm at Blue C Sushi in Fremont on Tuesday or Friday or Monday and an endless chain of sushi boats floats by on a waterway that circles back on itself over and over again. I look at the watch every day for a year and a half before the water inside evaporates, bouncing back and forth between where I was, where I am, and where I'm going. I understand that they're all related, but not in the way the hands of the watch suggest.

I write 3,000 words for a magazine and the editor tells me it's garbage because it isn't linear and I use too many metaphors. I look at my watch and try to explain that the paragraphs jump from past to present to future because time isn't linear. Life happens all at once, moment by moment. I ask myself if I'm still taking the medications that make me sane because this all sounds a bit manic and the editor stares at me like I am either a raven or a writing desk and tells me I've wasted his time and asks me to leave. Eighteen years later I'll write 3,155 more words in a book about my life and see how the minutes of then are now.

13

Lying to ourselves is more deeply ingrained

than lying to others.

—Fyodor Dostoevsky

I'm eight and my brother is ten and unlike him, I hate to read because I prefer listening and looking at pictures. I despise reading so much that Mom and Dad bribe me at a rate of three cents a page. Hardy Boys mysteries: *The House on the Cliff. While the Clock Ticked. The Secret of the Caves.* I always count the pages and do the multiplication before starting anything. I want chapter books because they're the longest, which means I'll be rich.

I "finish" a book in record time and Dad doesn't trust that I can read so quickly. He quizzes me by opening to a page and asking a question. I've failed this test before and now game the system by opening the books to a handful of places, pressing them hard, facedown, and creasing the spine. I read a few pages before and after each crease and when they magically open to just the right spot, I have all the answers. I'm developing a talent for deception. I owe my parents money.

People are exceptional liars. As it turns out, lying is a highly sophisticated process and demands a huge amount of energy in the brain, not to mention the emotional energy of keeping a secret. Dishonesty in humans likely evolved as a survival tactic. We lie for gain, for acceptance, to protect against loss, and because "Yes, your ass does look terrible in those pants" is not a pleasant way to start a date.

We learn to fake-cry at age one and start lying at about three, and we lie to others and our pets and teddy bears. And, perhaps most fascinating and impactful, we lie to ourselves. We're motivated to create and see the world in ways that support how we want to see ourselves and how we want the world to see us in it. The more we believe in self-deception, the easier it becomes to convince others of it. And that can shape reality.

But when we lie too much, we build a world that demands secrets and secrets are stressful. Beyond that, we erode trust, which impacts self-esteem because the world stops believing us even when we're telling the truth. Sometimes we course-correct. Other times we double down. When it comes to self-deception, sometimes we're simply blind in order to survive.

Some books I like. Dad has piles of mountain literature that take up most of the white shelves in the staircase that leads to their bedroom. Some are first editions with eroding, threadbare spines and have pages that fall out. Others are enormous picture books with titles like *Mountains of the Middle Kingdom* and *The Himalaya* and *Everest, the West Ridge*. But he chooses a small book and tells me, "I think you'll like this," and hands me *Banner in the Sky* by James Ramsey Ullman. It's 288 pages, by far the longest book I've ever read, and I say, "But there are no pictures . . ."

Set in the late nineteenth century, it's the fictional story of a Swiss boy named Rudi who's drawn to the last great challenge of the Alps, the Citadel, the same mountain that killed his father. I dive into a world of sharp mountains, blue smears of ice, gray stone that falls at random, near misses, tragedy, obstacles, doubt, and triumph. It is the hero's journey. I ignore homework and lie about it because I'm devouring the pages. I read at recess and lunch and hide the book in class and turn my light back on after bedtime when I'm sure Mom and Dad are asleep.

When I hand the bent pages back to Dad three days later, he looks very skeptical, which isn't uncommon because he's a skeptic and I've been known to lie.

But tonight there's no deceit and Dad flips to a page and asks, "How did Rudi get the man out of the crevasse?"

"He tied his clothes together and lowered his walking staff."

Dad doesn't say anything but smiles.

"Why did Captain Winter pummel Rudi after he just saved his life?"

This is harder and I have to think because I barely know what *pummel* means and it doesn't make sense that someone would punch a person who just saved them. Dad waits and looks over the top of the book until I concede. "Rudi was nearly naked and had been lying on the snow," he tells me. "He was hypothermic, which is when your body gets too cold and all the blood leaves your extremities and goes inside and fills all your guts to keep them alive. And when it's really bad, sometimes the best way to get the blood flowing back through your limbs is to beat the be-jeezus out of them." This is one of Dad's words that I love most: bejeezus.

I say, "One more." Dad flips through a few pages and reads to himself. He reads another page and smiles. "Captain Winter tells Rudi something about being young . . ."

"The part about chocolate?"

"No," Dad says. "Something else. Youth is the time for what?"

"Dreams!"

Dad closes the book and says, "Indeed." And pays me $8.64. When Mom asks me if I spent it on candy, I lie.

I'm twenty-four. It's 7 P.M. and dark and drizzly as I thumb through my old copy of *Banner in the Sky*, parked in a mostly empty lot at the Canadian border. My phone buzzes and the text message reads, "30 minutes out."

The streetlights collect as a thousand orange drops on my windshield and they are my memories of four years in Seattle. I think of all the late nights in Barb's studio and the early mornings climbing. Seattle is where I've crafted and solidified my nascent identity of photographer. I have climbed, made art, and fallen in love. When the love dried up, I decided to move away.

The girl who taught me about heartbreak was named Gail. She was an acupuncturist with olive skin and arms and legs that were muscular and feminine at the same time. She had round, cute features with very white teeth and a bit of an overbite from sucking her thumb for too long as a child. Because she was eight years older than me, Gail taught me many things before we said goodbye after two years. Here is a short list:

1. Kale grows best in full sunlight.
2. In traditional Chinese medicine, the body has twelve main meridians.
3. Being late is always disrespectful unless your plane crashed or someone is dead.
4. When it comes to oral sex, if my face doesn't look like a glazed donut, I'm not doing it right.
5. Don't lie.
6. A futon mattress on the floor is not a bed.

Gail had a bed. A real bed. Just after we split up (because I was always late and a bit of a liar), I made a bed frame and bought a mattress because I didn't know what else to do. I slept six hours over five days, living in my friend's family garage sawing, sweating, sanding, and swearing a bed into existence. Mom asked, "Are you taking your pills?" and I could hear one therapist or another say something about mania. I've always worked in manic spurts, trying to create my way out of turmoil. Plus, I thought maybe if I had a bed Gail might love me again. She didn't.

In Seattle, I climbed mostly with Jesse Huey and Shane Chelone. We had done as many big routes on as many of the Cascades volcanoes as we were ready for. I took pictures and got better at composition and light. Jesse loved climbing. Shane and I loved to talk about climbing. I preferred the stories to the act, but I had to collect them for myself. We ran countless miles, trained in the rain, and slept in parking lots. When the police told us we weren't allowed to sleep at Walmart and asked if they could search our car, I could see their disappointment picking through dirty socks, stinky long underwear, wet boots, and ropes. "What's this stuff?" they asked, as if we might be tying people up, stealing their clothes, and killing them with our ice axes.

We talked endlessly of climbing and our heroes like Steve House and Conrad Anker and Barry Blanchard and Jimmy Chin and Dean Potter, retelling their tales as if they were our own, imagining ourselves as much better than we were. Whenever I told my stories to girls at bars, the mountains were much bigger and the routes twice as hard and I grew two inches. One climber who will remain nameless liked to say, "If the women could see us now, we'd be knee deep in pussy!" which turned out to be a lie. I discovered that most girls weren't really interested in climbing but liked climbers because they have unkempt hair and muscles.

I think of these things while staring through the dots on my windshield with *Banner in the Sky* forgotten in my lap because I can't focus on anything for long unless I'm heartbroken and making furniture.

Steve Swenson calls and says, "I'm almost there." I look over my shoulder across the parking lot.

"Okay. Just look for the U-Haul." The trailer's so heavy the rear bumper is within inches of the pavement, making the car look like it might spontaneously pop into a wheelie at any moment. Even if the lot was full, I'd be impossible to miss.

Steve is fifty and sturdy with a hooked nose and dark hair, thick eyebrows, and looks like Commander Spock's cousin. He has lean muscles and powerful calves and thighs, and I have known him since I was eight years old. He's what might be called a climber's climber, a "dark horse," an athlete revered within the community but faceless and nameless to the world outside of climbing. He's humble and confident, modest but opinionated about this sport and all other things. His wife, Ann, is a librarian and a quiet anchor to his relentlessness. She's kind, compassionate, and motherly.

I wonder why all government buildings make you feel like you're a criminal as we walk into the linoleum waiting room of the immigration office. Steve hands the border agent our passports and the deed to their new house near Banff, Alberta, and tells the man he's an engineer and a climber. There's only one answer when someone declares themselves a climber to the uninitiated.

"What's the highest mountain you've ever climbed?" the agent asks.

"Everest." Steve doesn't look up from the form he's filling out.

"Okay, what's the second-highest mountain you've ever climbed?"

"K2," Steve answers flatly. I'm invisible watching the exchange and notice the agent's sideways smile.

"But you used oxygen on both, right?"

Steve signs his name on the last line, looks up as he slides the papers across, and says, "Neither."

"And who are you and why are you driving *his* things to *his* new home?" The agent seems far less impressed with me and my unkempt hair.

"I'm just a friend and I need some extra cash and Steve has to work."

"How long will you be in Canada?"

"Seven days." This is a lie. I'll live in Steve's house for four years.

The Canadian Rockies are the epicenter of the hardest alpine climbing in North America outside of Alaska. It's also not a place I can legally work, so I'll be forced to make money from photography. Mom will beg me to get a job as a bartender or server but I'll argue fanatically and tell her that would be the death of my dreams. Steve understands my zeal and Ann is overflowing with patience. Together they have the understanding for everything that comes with being me and their home will become the launchpad of my future.

I'll be an illegal alien and leave no paper trail. I'm a gleeful and unapologetic criminal and will feel no guilt for this transgression. Ever. I would pursue climbing and photography at any cost.

I'm sweating as I follow Eamonn Walsh and Raphael Slawinksi to the bottom of a funnel of ice that climbs to a hanging snowfield and another pillar of frozen water above. My boots are laced low and loose, the way I've learned, and I listen to our breathing over a low rumble of snow falling down the climb in miniature avalanches. We call these mini slides "spindrift," and I know today is likely to be wet and my collar will be constantly packed with loose snow. When we get to the bottom of the funnel, the spindrift is nearly constant and I wonder if climbing is wise. But

Raph and Eamonn are putting on their harnesses, so I don't say anything because I don't want to appear scared, even though I am.

Raph is long and lean and moves more like a dancer than a climber. In a sport that is often brutish, he's graceful and delicate, nearly silent, and unafraid because he's a physicist and calculates mathematical risk to override fear. Eamonn is huge. His biceps are bigger than my thighs and he talks in a low, lumbering voice that makes him sound humble despite anything he might be saying. He's bold like Raph but probably wiser because he uses intuition as much as math to manage risk.

Raph launches up the ice trailing two ropes, one for Eamonn and another for me, and we start climbing together when the ropes become tight. Climbing continuously as a single team is called simul climbing and comes with the added benefit of speed but the danger of pulling everyone off if anyone falls.

The ice above us climbs a narrow runnel and we're stacked on top of each other as the little avalanches become bigger until there's a constant stream of white that makes it impossible to see, impossible to look up, and finally impossible to move. When a break comes, Eamonn and I sprint upward while Raph makes slow progress through the steep, loose snow above.

Long loops of rope hang below Eamonn and me when we arrive at the bottom of the snowfield. Raph is 100 feet ahead, wading through thigh-high snow and grunting. Eamonn steps out of the funnel and secures himself to the rock while I fidget with my zipper and try to empty all the packed snow from my collar. But before I can secure myself next to him, a small wall of spindrift knocks my feet out from under me. I grab blindly for my axes and my lips form the most perfect O. But before I can summon the letter *F*, my mouth fills with snow and I get washed back down the climb.

It's chaotic and loud and my ears are full of white noise. Nylon is tearing. Metal is scraping. Ice and stone are falling around me as I'm weightless for 75 feet, falling backward down the vertical funnel we just climbed. When the rope finally catches me, I'm dangling limp, folded in half backward and upside down while the spindrift continues to fill up my nose and open mouth, which is still trying to find the letter *F.*

When it all stops, I claw for the rock and swing my axes and try to kick my feet into the ice, but one ankle is Jell-O and lifeless and just flops off no matter how hard I kick. There's no pain but I know that it's either broken or the ligaments are torn or both. I start doing pull-ups with my axes and climbing with one foot. My thumb is throbbing and stinging and I taste blood. I keep pulling myself up and breathing as more spindrift pours over the edge while Eamonn says something, but I can't hear him.

Back at the bottom of the snowfield, I'm dry-heaving with a cut lip and a sprained hand and one working foot. "I think we should go down." Honesty is easy when it's the last choice you have.

We make crutches from ski poles, but it's usually easier to crawl or slide, and Raph and Eamonn watch me and laugh in the way you do when things have gone very wrong.

My clothes are soaked as I crawl into the back of the car and try to take the boot off my ankle, which looks a bit like a grapefruit. Raph drives to a gas station and buys me a six-pack of Corona and ibuprofen as all the pain seeps in. The world hurts and I notice every bump, bounce, and crack in the road.

"You've had a good fall." The doctor has a penchant for understatement.

"Yeah, about a hundred feet." Stories grow quickly.

There are no broken bones but all my ligaments are torn. He gives me a boot and some pills and asks if I have insurance. I lie and say I do. He sends me home and says to look for the bill in the mail. I won't.

It's easier to sit on the floor to get undressed as I strip the layers off my torso and push my long underwear over my knees and down my calves until a searing pain stops me. At some point during the fall, a spike from my crampon punctured my leg, leaving a deep hole in my calf. Small pieces of fat and muscle have dried to the fabric and are getting pulled from the hole. I wad up my shirt and bite down and peel the flesh and fabric apart.

Finally, my long underwear is around my ankles and I'm naked, picking small black fibers from the wound and tucking the dangly bits back into the hole and laugh-crying as I crawl into the bathtub. I tip my head back and Eamonn calls, "You all right?"

I'm a little drunk and the painkillers are starting to work.

"Yeah, I'm fine." It's another lie.

To the oldest part of our brain, the experience of climbing is interpreted as an act of survival and survival is stressful work. The sympathetic nervous system fires up and we step into fight, flight, or freeze and choose to fight. We fight gravity. We fight fear. We fight with our muscles and every cell of our body. We fight with our conscious and subconscious minds alike and the whole game is learning to manage the stress response and ultimately work in tandem with our brain and body in pursuit of a goal. In that way, it becomes an act of mindfulness because in order to survive, we're forced to distill order from chaos and focus on the now. The discomfort of it all is offset by the highs that come with it. It's beautiful and breathtaking and life-affirming in a way that few other sports can ever be. The conscious mind colors the experience with all sorts of stories and little self-deceptions about what we're doing and why. But to the ancient part of the brain, it's all the same thing; in that five-hundred-million-year-old piece of the mind, there is no poetry or story and we can tell no lies to escape the fact that the neurobiological basis of climbing is simple: Don't die.

Chaos is what I know best.

When am I going to get in another fight? When is the next conflict? The next punch? The next therapist? I'm at home. Now I'm in treatment. Now I'm homeless. Now I'm in a new home. Now I'm back home.

Some variance in our developmental years isn't a bad thing because it teaches adaptability, resilience, and independence. But when that's taken too far, maladaptive strategies develop in order to correct for emotional instability, and quite often we lie to ourselves about what we're doing and why. We lie to support stories that drive action that reinforces the deepest understanding of ourselves, and risk is a common manifestation.

There is a direct correlation between certain mental afflictions (including bipolar), children who experience abundant toxic stress, and tolerance *for* and the pursuit *of* risk. Risk is all about survival and that is the world we know. We learned that forecasting the future is usually wasted effort. We think less of potential negative consequences and exchange stability for an immediate experience at all costs. It doesn't make sense to invest in the long game because everything is always changing, so we choose to live fast and hard and think little of the delayed benefits and harms because risk-taking gives us what we want now. If there is no tomorrow, my brain says, try anything. Fuck it.

Two months later I take another enormous fall and puncture the opposite leg. It's clear to everyone else that my ambition often outpaces my judgment and always outpaces my skill. But I'm a master of self-deception. I'm not careless but I'm not careful either and a habit of falling in the mountains never really ends well. But I keep climbing and taking pictures and more of my heroes become my friends and climbing partners. In time, I lie less about my experience because I'm amassing more, even when I fall. Especially then. All my heroes have war stories and I'm busy making my own.

Most days pass safely because I'm lucky and climb with the best. They know that pictures in magazines and advertisements are good for them and their climbing careers, and together maybe we can make enough money to go on more trips to increasingly bigger mountains. That is how this goes. Some girls at the bars even know my name now and I love this. I'm a humming ball of exuberance, scars, and outsized confidence. Life feels like a long tennis volley as I bounce from car to climb to camera.

Eamonn and Raph and I find an untouched piece of mountain on the north face of Mount Bryce via a steep but easy couloir with short steps of ice. We climb it in a short, uneventful day.

I climb the north face of Snow Dome with Dana Ruddy and Ian Welsted. The line ascends almost 2,000 feet of smeared ice but we stop 60 feet short of the summit under an enormous hanging ice cliff. When night catches up, we chop a ledge behind a frozen pillar and hope the ice cliff above doesn't break off in the night and sweep us away. We call it a first ascent despite the final 60 feet and some people disagree, but I reject their objections. We name the climb "Polarity" as a play on "*polar*" and the oscillation of our minds between elation and terror. On these days, I love climbing.

I have a love affair with a girl named Suzy and she dies in an avalanche. I don't know how to feel or if I feel anything at all and I skip the funeral.

Freddie Wilkinson, Kevin Mahoney, and I are climbing the Grand Central Couloir on Mount Kitchener but get off route, which saves our lives when an avalanche sweeps down the chute and erases everything in its path. The mountain shakes and booms as rocks fall and we look at each other and, of course, laugh. Survival stories sell and I'm surviving. I sell more pictures.

An acquaintance from Seattle rappels off the end of a rope in Alaska and dies. On these days I hate climbing, but I never admit it.

The Mediterranean is clear and blue and stretches out peacefully 50 feet below me and I am taking pictures of Sonnie Trotter climbing ropeless when the limestone my rope is anchored to breaks and I'm upside down again and very wet as I cannonball into the sea. The rope pulls the broken rock down with it and it splashes into the water a few feet from my head and begins to sink. I am tied to it, getting more and more tangled and trying, ridiculously, to hold my camera above my head. I manage to un-clip myself from everything and swim to the shore, all the while holding the camera above the water. Somewhere in my memory Mom says, "Cory, you are so stubborn!" and she's right. I look like a wet dog and pretend I'm not shaken, but it is a lie.

Sonnie loans me his camera and I make a picture of him sus-pended from the peak of a high arch over frothy water and sell it to his sponsor for the cover of their spring catalog and buy a new camera and call the trip a wash. Breaking even is better than drowning.

I drive seventeen hours straight and use coffee to swallow caffeine pills and the bottle tells me to "Win Your Day." Dim lights of interstate towns rush by and my check engine light is on and never goes off. I listen to heavy, aggressive hip-hop. Hip-hop is outright mastery of the English language and I respect it even though it feels like it's not entirely mine. When I get to Yosemite, my whole body is tingling. I have sunflower seeds and beef jerky stuck in my teeth and it tastes like a cat shit in my mouth.

Two days later Alex Honnold is climbing a crack 3,000 feet above the valley floor high on El Capitan. The sun is setting and darkness is creeping up the wall, making the space below him black and his shadow long. He climbs easily and asks me if I'd like him to do it again while I hang in space and spin and hope the stone doesn't break because there is no water below me. I take a picture as he moves from one hold to the next. His hand is blurry, but the shadow of it is defined, and I think it's strange how motion and stillness can coexist, how fast our minds can go even while we're standing still.

I get on a plane to Seattle and have a panic attack because I live on caffeine and very little sleep these days. A new psychiatrist gives me diazepam and I nibble half pills before climbs and on flights and after particularly heavy nights of drinking when I'm stricken with anxiety. I take antidepressants and mood stabilizers and benzos to keep me calm and level. I drink caffeine to counteract the lethargy and alcohol to calm the caffeine and inhale nicotine to calm my nerves on ledges that are overhung with ice, and I don't see it as a problem because I don't see it all. Lack of awareness is its own form of self-deception.

It's a beautiful time but everything is moving so fast that I forget to be grateful. It's all blurry and the only things that stand still are the pictures of moments I freeze but never see. I will forget most of it because the world is in constant motion and, in my mind, it's time to slam my foot against the accelerator and speed up. It's time to let grit overtake me, to be relentlessness. To grind. I tell myself I'm not a talented climber and that my pictures aren't groundbreaking. Sometimes I hate it all. But sometimes I love it more than anything. I'll hang in that space for years, spinning on the end of a rope high above everything or tangled in it while I sink. Bigger. Better. Faster. More. I have momentum and hope and youth is the time for dreams, so I dream harder. It's time to move on to bigger mountains.

Not all high-risk behavior is maladaptive and none of this is to say that climbing is bad or that everyone who does it is chasing and running from pieces of themselves. Many are adding pieces and I'm doing the same. I'm only exploring me and my head. Some people do it to be in nature and some do it for a little adrenaline buzz and some people just love the movement and the places you end up. I love all those things too, but that love comes from a different place. And besides, climbing is healthier than heroin. But for *me* to think that all the speed and falls and near misses and death, emotion, stimulation, and risk that swarm around me aren't tied to the way my brain is wired? That's just another lie. I'll have to see death up close before I understand the game I'm playing. I find it in Peru.

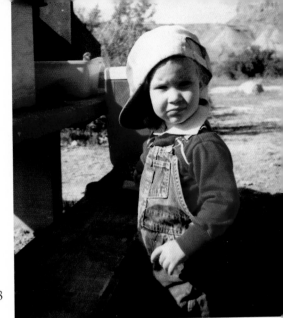

Camping in southern Utah, 1983

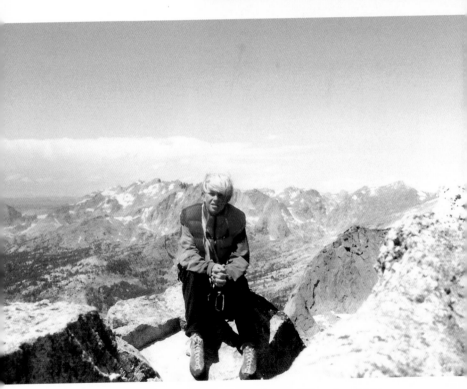

On the summit of Pingora, Wind River Range, Wyoming, 1993

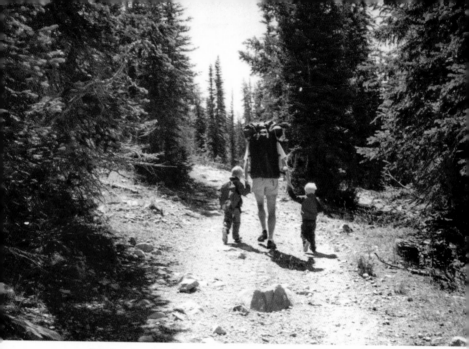

My brother, Dad, and me backpacking in the Uintas, Utah, 1984

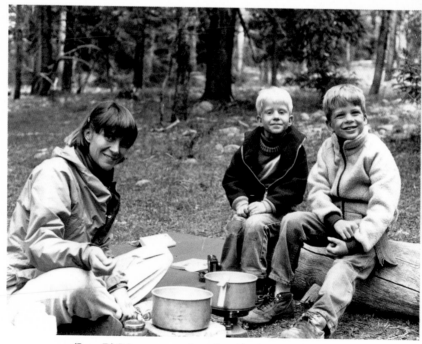

(L to R) Mom, me, and my brother backpacking, 1986

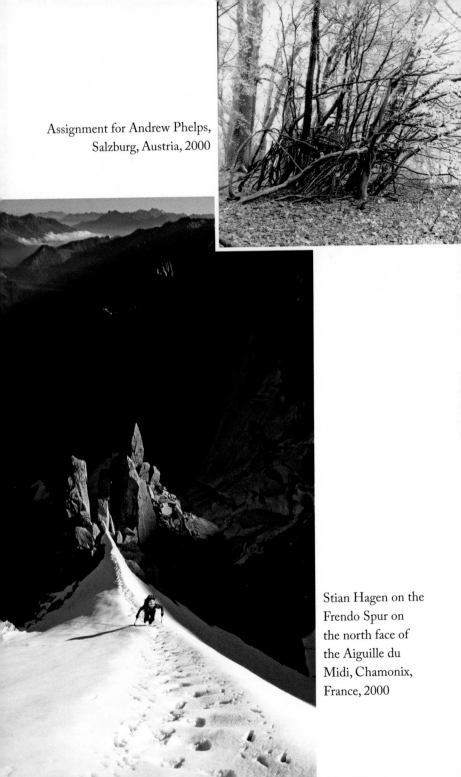

Assignment for Andrew Phelps,
Salzburg, Austria, 2000

Stian Hagen on the
Frendo Spur on
the north face of
the Aiguille du
Midi, Chamonix,
France, 2000

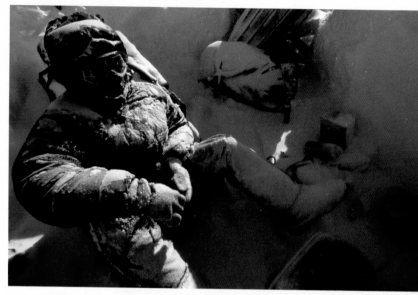

Dave Garrow on Mt. Logan, Yukon Territories, Canada, 2003

Homeless woman, Seattle, 2001

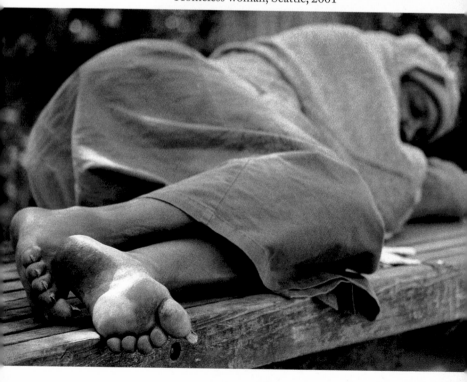

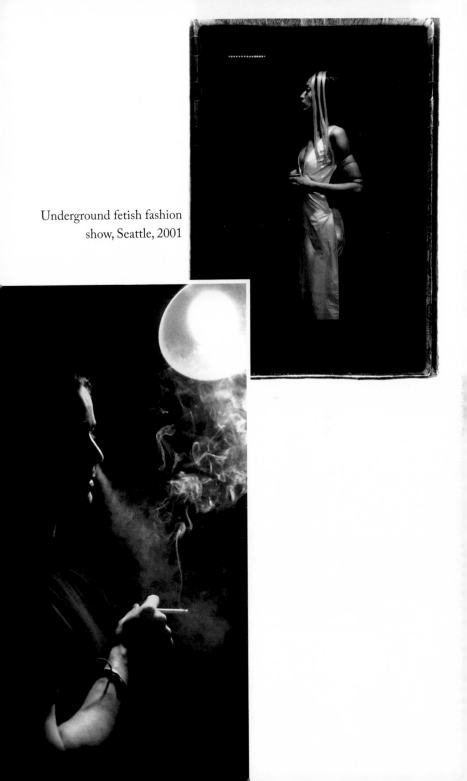

Underground fetish fashion
show, Seattle, 2001

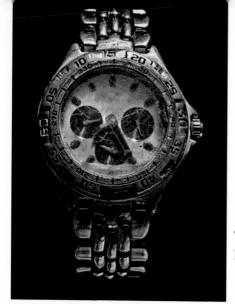

The watch after returning
home from Australia

A Peruvian girl crosses the street in Huaraz, Peru, 2006

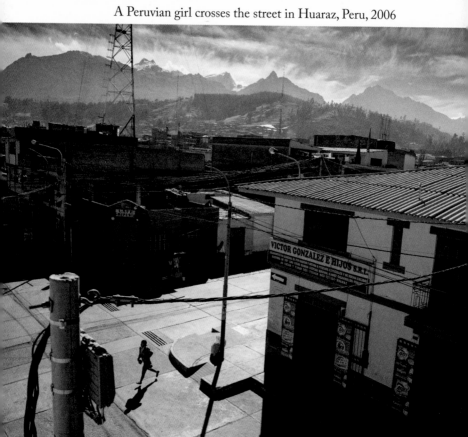

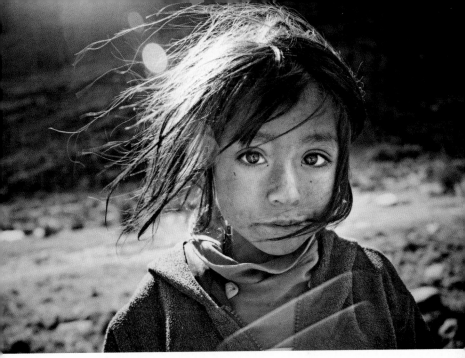

Quechua girl, Santa Cruz Valley, Peru, 2006

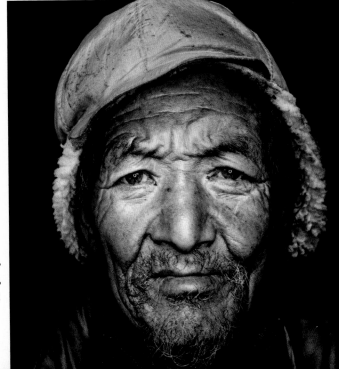

Hermitage keeper,
Khumbu Valley,
Nepal, 2008

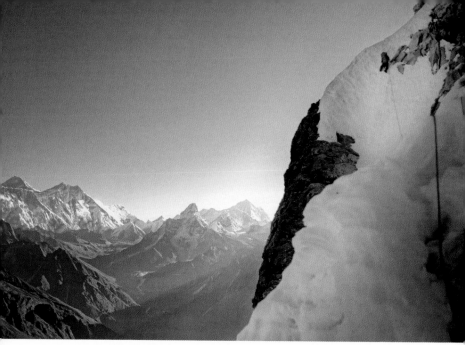

Ines Papert traverses the north face of Kwangde Shar on the first ascent of Cobra Norte with the Khumbu Valley below. In the distance rise Everest, Lhotse, Ama Dablam, and Makalu (L to R)

Kevin Mahoney (R) and Freddie Wilkinson (L), Nuptse, Nepal, 2009

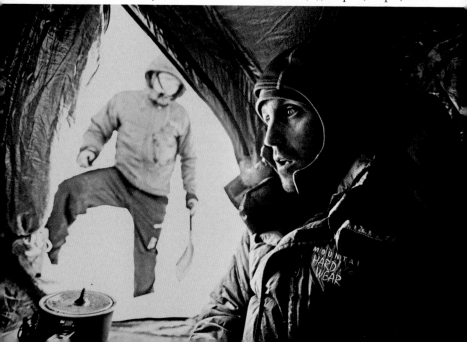

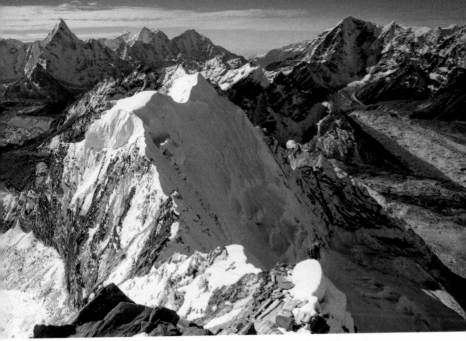

Freddie Wilkinson on the West Ridge of Nuptse, Nepal, 2009

Tea time with Pakistani army officers, Karakorum Himalaya, winter, 2010

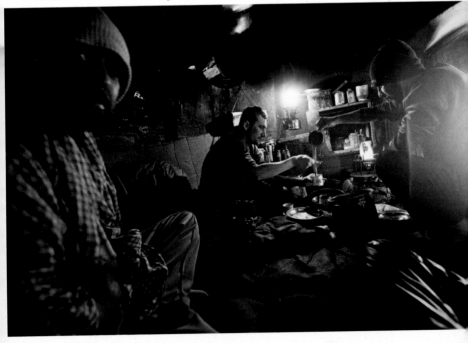

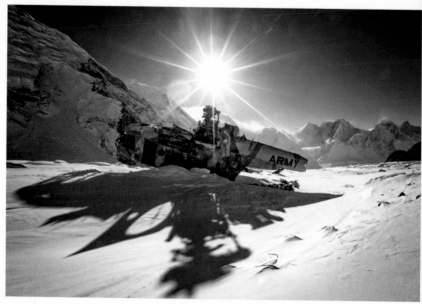

Pakistani army helicopter near Gasherbrum II base camp,
Karakorum Himalaya, winter, 2010

Denis Urubko (R) and Simone Moro (L) climb into the sun on summit day of
the first winter ascent of Gasherbrum II, 8,035 meters (26,362 feet)

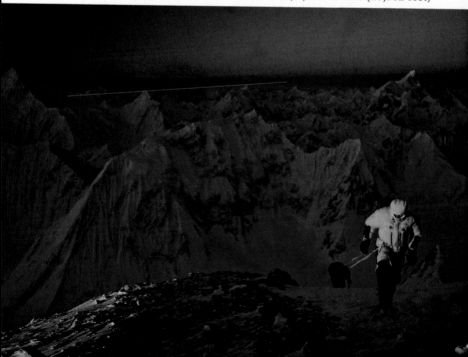

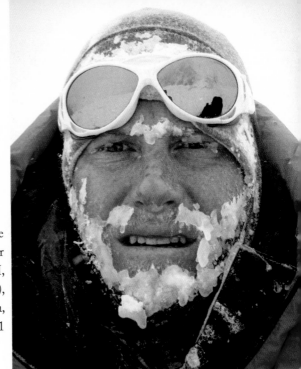

Self-portrait after the avalanche; first winter ascent of Gasherbrum II, 8,035 meters (26,362 feet), Karakorum Himalaya, Pakistan, February 4, 2011

Matt Segal climbs into an ancient cave complex below the village of Tsele, Mustang, Nepal, 2011

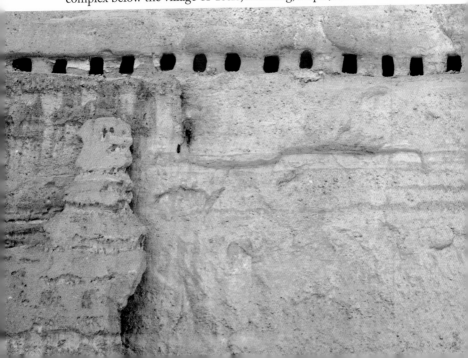

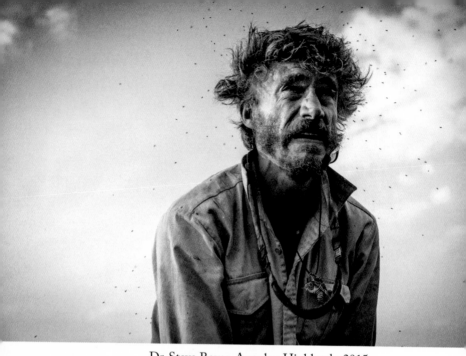

Dr. Steve Boyes, Angolan Highlands, 2015

Polar bear on Rudolph Island, Franz Josef Land, Russia, 2013

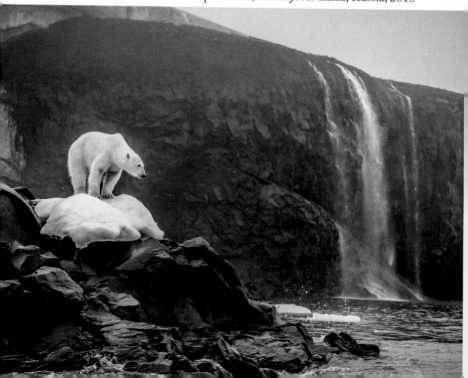

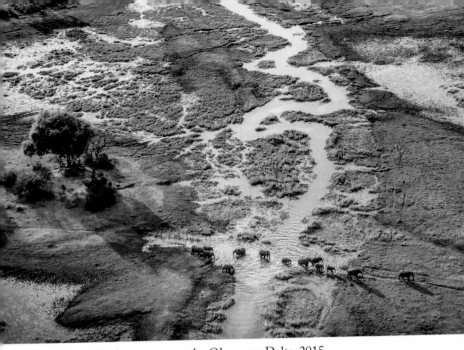

Elephants traverse the Okavango Delta, 2015

Sunset in the Angolan Highlands, 2015

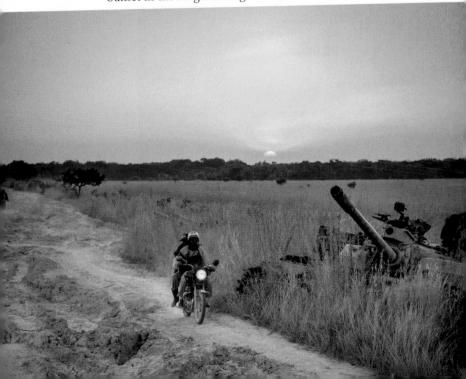

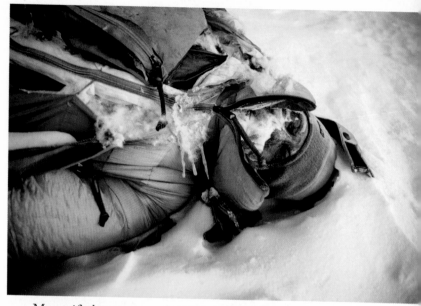

Mummified corpse around 8,000 meters (26,240 feet) on Lhotse, 2010

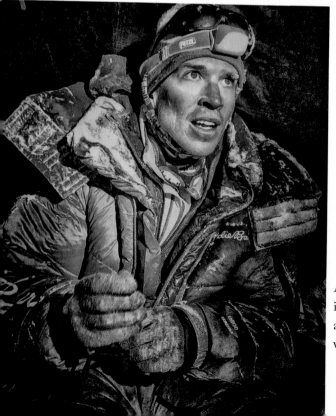

Adrian Ballinger back in advanced base camp after climbing Everest without oxygen, 2017

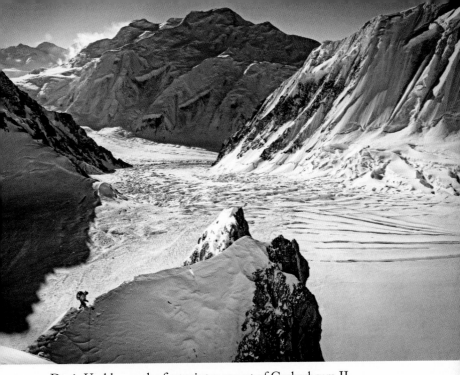

Denis Urubko on the first winter ascent of Gasherbrum II,
Karakorum Himalaya, Pakistan, 2011

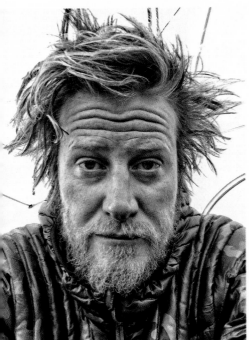

Me forty hours without
sleep back in advanced base
camp after climbing Everest
without oxygen, 2016

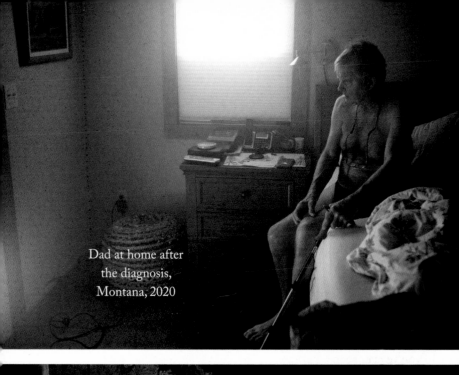

Dad at home after
the diagnosis,
Montana, 2020

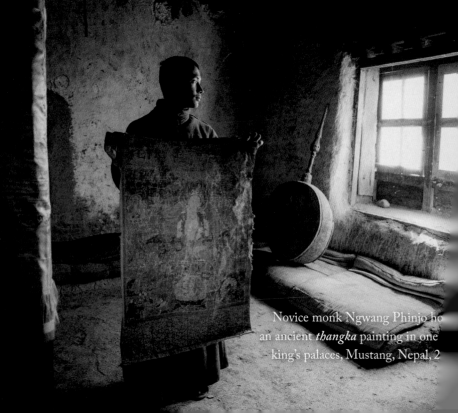

Novice monk Ngwang Phinjo ho
an ancient *thangka* painting in one
king's palaces, Mustang, Nepal, 2

14

The man who runs away may fight again.

—DEMOSTHENES

I f you've ever seen a Paramount movie, you'll recognize a 19,762-foot mountain with a halo of stars bending neatly over the summit. Viewed from the northern slope of the Santa Cruz Valley in the Cordillera Blanca of Peru, Artesonraju is one of the most symmetrical peaks in the world. But now, from the valley floor, it appears as a nearly formless black ghost silhouetted against a navy sky. Until the moon rises at 2:31 A.M., it will remain an apparition, shadowed by its own mass. The twenty-two neatly placed stars are conspicuously absent, replaced by a million tiny pinholes.

I prepare to leave base camp at 9:30 P.M. and tell my teammates that I'll be back in no more than a day as I test the small two-way radios and agree to check in every two hours. In one of my mercurial, angst-filled episodes of being motivated and twenty-five, I've decided to climb the northeast face of Artesonraju alone.

The Cordillera Blanca is the highest mountain range outside of the Himalaya, with peaks as high as 22,200 feet. Like it was for so many ambitious climbers before me, the Blanca will be my springboard to the Himalaya. But that will take two more years and many more nights that begin just like this.

I turn my headlamp on low and traverse the swampy meadow on the south side of camp, jumping from tuft to tuft, trying to keep my socks dry. But just before I reach the northern flank, I plunge my right foot into a muddy soup that drenches me to the knee.

My camera bounces off my right hip bone and I'm angry at it the way you're angry at whatever you just hit your head on even though the thing did nothing wrong. I wonder why I have it with me aside from the fact that it's a part of my costume. I want something more from photography and question if I should keep climbing just for me. I also know that climbing is what opens the door to photography, but I don't want my images to be just rock and ice and climbers. I want to expand beyond this world, and I fear I might have accidentally chained my voice with a very short tether. I'm sure I will never fully escape the adventure trope. These are the thoughts I think walking alone at night, asking my brain if it might shut the fuck up for a minute or two, and it says no. I keep walking.

I enter the forest and leave a track of single wet footprints. The limbs of shrubby trees appear as a tangle of sinewy arms hugging me in the low canopy. Sweat begins to saturate my layers as my scent mixes with the dust and sweet pollen trapped by the leaves and moisture of the valley bottom. As the pitch steepens, the trees give way to loose, rocky terrain covered by a thin layer of moss and yellow grass and my ankles flex and bend as I step in dark shadows.

I reach the top of the stones just after midnight and turn the light to its brightest and study the granite slabs that separate me from the bottom of the snow. A waterfall flows from the underside of a large hanging glacier and sends boulders and chunks of ice crashing off the slabs to my left and I think the mountains are awfully loud. I shed my wet shirt and a layer of steam rises off my skin into the bright headlamp beam and obscures my view. I switch it off and the darkness of the mountain overwhelms me while I listen to the creaks and cracks of the glacier overhead.

After I spend another hour connecting ledges in a chaotic zig-zag, the mountain has overtaken the horizon and disappeared altogether. All I can see is the circle of light at my feet and I am an island. I think I'm always an island.

Four hours after leaving base camp, I pull my ice axes from my back and plant the picks in the snow and pull on my harness and crampons and a pair of dry socks and another dry shirt. I secure a short length of rope in a coil over my neck and look up the slope until the light fades into a black question mark.

Three years from now, in 2009, Andre Agassi will write that tennis is the loneliest sport. When I read the words, I remember this night and know he never climbed a mountain alone, in darkness, untethered to anything other than several centimeters of dull steel dug precariously into brittle ice. I look down and kick my feet into the slope, but I can't see because my camera is casting a shadow and I am annoyed by it again.

Agassi will describe staring down an opponent but never touching them and I will think of this moment, staring into an infinite darkness framed by my feet and yawning with gravity as my muscles fatigue and lungs gasp for too-thin air. If there is an opponent at all in solo climbing, it's an uncaring and indifferent piece of earth that is constantly throwing rocks at you while you dodge avalanches and storms, head bowed in concentration and praying to a God you only believe in when you're terrified. Most often the opponent is yourself and your own fear. Tennis is not the loneliest sport.

The scraps of metal shake under the weight of my body, threatening to skate out at any moment and send my soft frame toma-hawking down thousands of feet while my arms and legs are ripped from their joints and my head explodes. There is nothing to stop me if I fall.

They will find my body in a colorful, contorted heap that looks like an unsolved Rubik's Cube, and everyone will be sad. My parents will fly to Peru and meet with my climbing partners and find a way to cremate me and I'll fly home with them, tucked neatly in Mom's carry-on. Mom and Dad will gather everyone in a field and they'll all have a tiny pile of pale ash in their hands and release me into the sky. They'll wipe their hands on their pants and I'll leave chalky stains. This is how I will die and become just a picture on a wall.

After 300 feet of climbing I scan the slope above, angling up and left to follow the contours of a dark rib of stone. On the edge of the light I see a patch of red that I dismiss as trash from a previous ascent and keep climbing. After another 50 feet the scrap seems too big to be garbage and I kick and stab faster until I reach the huddled clump. Whatever it is, it's trapped between the rock and ice, and I'm confused by what I'm looking at. Pieces of metal and nylon sit in a tangled mess. There's a red jacket and an ice axe broken at the hilt. There is a backpack and a confusing harness with a metal bar and the pieces come together all at once as I stare at the lifeless body.

According to some studies, humans can experience twenty-seven distinct emotions. In moments of shock those emotions can overlap and blend, becoming unidentifiable and overwhelming. Fear. Confusion. Awe. Excitement. Anxiety. Entrancement. The brain has a hard time distinguishing which is which because different experiences carry different triggers and it can take minutes, days, even years to unravel and identify. The sympathetic nervous system overrides rational thinking and behavior and we're often left with an irrational response.

I'm alone, high on a mountain in darkness, staring at a corpse.

My brain does what it likes to do and organizes horror into humor, and I radio base camp and whisper, "I see dead people. . . ."

Someone says, "Take lots of pictures," and I say, "No shit," and another person tells me to look for identification, and someone else says, "Is there any way to get, like, something for DNA?" because none of us have ever dealt with this before and they are as lost as I am.

The body is old and decomposed. The legs are mostly missing and the arms are empty red sleeves and I can't see the head. I untangle the mess of cord and free the broken axe as the dead, organic weight resists my attempts to pull it from the ice. I jerk the torso upright and it breaks free and flips backward revealing a dark hole into the chest cavity where the head used to be. That this is—was—a human is nearly incomprehensible.

I take pictures and search the pockets for ID and find none. DNA is probably useless but as good an idea as any and so I pull a Ziploc bag of nuts from my jacket and dump it out. The peanuts and cashews and Brazil nuts bounce down the ice and out of sight while I put on a glove and shine my headlamp into the hole where the head should be. I shove my hand in and search for anything solid. It's mostly frozen but a bit mushy and mostly empty and I scrape my fingers along what I think is the rib cage.

In my hand there are two broken ribs and a long piece of collarbone covered in a gray-brown residue with larger, coagulated clumps of pulp that smear against the plastic bag as I tuck it into the top pocket of my pack next to the broken ice axe. I've lost my appetite for climbing. Tennis is definitely not the loneliest sport.

Back in town four days later, it's 8:30 A.M. and I'm eating a bun with unsalted butter and jam with two over-easy eggs on the roof of La Casa de Zarela. Huaraz stretches out in a patchwork of red-brick buildings with square rooftops that appear unfinished with long, uneven rebar jutting through concrete struts. In Peru, if there is exposed construction, you can claim the structure is unfinished and avoid property taxes. But to me, tax evasion looks like the remains of a bombed-out city with its bones reaching into the sky. There are large blue water tanks glaring in the sun and bedsheets and jeans and the occasional Quechua *jobona* hanging limp on clotheslines. Some roofs have grain laid out to dry and I watch people flip the laundry and thresh corn and collect water. I listen to a mixture of pigeons and dogs and horns, and it all appears muted and yellow through the dust.

Zarela has rented me a room in her personal apartment on the top floor of her hostel and being the roommate of the proprietor comes with special privileges. I can use the kitchen and I have my own key to come home late and drunk, occasionally with company. I'm also allowed to store human body parts in the freezer.

I pull the Ziploc out and place it in a bowl of hot water to thaw the scum off the bones before turning on the tap and watching it wash away. I have to mash some of the larger pieces through the drain screen with my fingers and it's hard to grasp what I'm doing. I've seen bodies in my life but holding the bones confuses my indifference with unease. I notice that they're smaller than I'd imagined ribs to be and have a smooth, coffee-yellow patina. I lay them on a towel and wonder what to do next.

I email a few pictures of the body to Will Gadd, the most connected and well known of my climbing friends, asking for help. He replies within minutes and tells me that the strange metal bar in the pictures is an old paragliding harness, which he knows because he's also a paraglider (he calls it "flying lawn chairs"). Because it's a world I know nothing of, Will writes a post with vague details on an international paragliding forum asking for any information anyone might have. Forty-eight hours later I open an email from a man named Klemen in Slovenia. The broken English reads:

This is my partner Marko. He disappears after paragliding from the summit. We lost him in the clouds and he never land. The mountain was too dangerous from that side with many avalanche and we never find any body.

The bones will be of no use because his name was Marko Azman and now I'm speaking with a woman named Daria from a stuffy internet café. She tells me her brother left for Peru in 1988 and never came home.

Daria peppers me with questions and asks for details while she translates for her parents. I stare blankly over the top of the plywood cubicle through a dusty window and read the words "Internet Café" backward and everything is a bit confusing.

Four days later I'm at the bus station helping Daria carry her duffel to a taxi, which is just a guy named Carlos making some extra cash on his lunch hour. Daria is athletic and has short brown hair. She wears wire-framed glasses and has all the angles of an Eastern European woman and smiles a lot. I wonder why because it seems this is a grim business.

We run errands in town and make a loose plan with a new friend named Brian who has agreed to help us. I've never ex-humed a body. Nor have I buried one. But the shopping list is short, and we buy a shovel and a digging bar and a pick, and commission a stone artisan to carve three small headstones with Marko's name and birth and death years on them. I will keep one and Daria another and we will leave one with him. We go to the open market, which smells of dead flesh and fresh produce. It's loud and stuffy as we weave between the stalls while people use rags to wave flies off the meat. We buy enough food for four days and have shoulder straps sewn onto a large black duffel and hope the body bag is big enough.

In another four days, Brian and I are traversing the same meadow and I manage to keep my feet dry. The orange trunks of the trees seem to lean in and form a tunnel specifically for this journey as we talk about climbing and mountains and death and girls. The dirt, dust, and sweat mix again into something salty and sweet and I wonder if the body will smell when we bring it down.

The slabs are easier to navigate in the light and we reach the bottom of the ice in three hours. The waterfall is louder in the heat of the day and small pebbles and pieces of ice rain down from the face, pelting our helmets and hands. I study the seracs overhead and am aware of what I was climbing under in darkness and wonder if Marko's death might have saved my life that night by stopping my climb. It is an unanswerable question.

We reach the body in fifteen minutes and make quick work of chopping the remains free and say things like "Sorry, Marko" while we load him into the duffel. It's too big. Marko has lost weight in the eighteen years he's been sitting on the mountain and his body is easier to fold than lay out. The remains sit too low in the body bag and it hangs below my waist, which makes downclimbing awkward. Brian reminds me not to fall and points out that the bag might be too big for Marko, but it's too small for both of us. I laugh but take his point.

Daria emerges from a blue tent and watches us traverse the meadow as the sun dips into the steep V of the valley and I notice how long our shadows are. I splash through mud because I no longer care if my feet are dry or wet and Marko is feeling heavy. The nylon is rubbing against my skin and cutting uneven, tender patches into my sunburned neck.

I remember my war literature class and Tim O'Brien's words: "They carried all they could bear, and then some, including a silent awe for the terrible power of the things they carried." This isn't war, but I understand a sliver of the verse as Daria helps lift the weight from my shoulders and I feel cool air rush across the sweat of my back.

After dark, the lantern smells like kerosene and burns with a low rumble while Brian and I listen to Daria dig through everything she remembers about Marko.

Like all memories, hers are a collage of sharp details that fray toward the edges, as if she is creating a portrait from torn-up pictures of the same face. There are very few shortcomings because she's learned what to keep and what to throw away. She cries as she resurrects her brother, who is lying silently in the duffel just outside the tent.

When I write this chapter in a café in Salzburg sixteen years later, I've known many people who have died climbing. I know that most of their last moments were spent in terror, and it haunts me. Some were dear friends and others I knew only briefly, but they were all kindred, and their names are Andre Callari and Rupert Rosedale. Micah Dash and Jonny Copp and Chhewang Nima Sherpa and Dean Potter. Scott Adamson and Kyle Dempster and Hayden Kennedy and Hansjörg Auer and Jess Roskelley and Ueli Steck and Hilaree Nelson and I'm sure that I have left others out.

Hayden lived with me for several seasons hanging Christmas lights for money and became one of the most talented climbers of a generation. After losing two close friends on a climb in Pakistan he wrote: "This is the painful reality of our sport, and I'm unsure what to make of it. Climbing is either a beautiful gift or a curse. . . . I see both light and dark."

Hayden took his own life hours after his fiancée was killed in an avalanche and I think this world is filled with unjust, poetic tragedy. Like him, I'm unsure of what to make of it. My mind is always full of words but there is nothing to say.

Words amidst tragedy rarely if ever touch the void of grief, let alone fill it. The need to speak is an attempt to bring something back . . . to undo something that can't be undone. And platitudes aren't all that comforting. Regardless, someone always says something like "*At least* they died doing what they loved." The search for a silver lining, the stumbling to make sense of death, doesn't make loss any less painful.

I read research papers and articles on grief and try to write a meaningful paragraph or two about neurobiology and stress hormones and try to sound smart. I try to unwind what happens in the brain because this is a book about mental health and this chapter seems important. Nothing comes out. Four stages. Seven stages. Science is another incomplete language for something that sits beyond words. And still, say what you can and mean what you say and when there are no more words just let the silence speak. For a moment, let the silence scream.

The words that really matter in the wake of passing are the stories we tell of our loved ones. Stories fill up the space they leave behind and we can see their faces and hear their laugh and reach into something shapeless and touch them. So long as we tell stories, they can never really die.

In the morning I help Daria shoulder the body and Brian and I gather the shovel and pick and make our way to a collection of sharp granite boulders. Daria wanders back and forth across the rocky terrace looking at the ground and then up and then down and then stops. She stands in silence for a moment before looking to us. "Here."

After three and a half hours there's a large pile of fresh dirt and roots and stones. I lean on the shovel with thick black sweat across my face and the crunch of dirt in my teeth. Daria lifts the bag and straddles the hole and lowers Marko into the ground, where he rests unevenly against the rocks that were too big to move. I think of sleeping under boulders and wish I could make his bed more comfortable but also think this is an appropriate place for a climber to sleep.

When all the dirt is filled in, I mix epoxy in a red bowl and brush it against a flat boulder. Daria sets the headstone in place, and I notice the dirt under her nails and in the creases of her fingers and clogging the pores of her delicate hands. I've never lost anyone this close to me. She has lost the same person twice and whispers something into the dirt.

It's late now and our shadows are long again. The grass is yellow and catches the sun in hot-white flashes. I'm very tired as I walk back across the field and my blistered hands ache from digging. Death is beautiful and terrible and living will kill you. I cry but the tears don't feel like mine.

Grief can be an astonishingly beautiful response to loss and the pain of it can stir a renewed appreciation for life. It makes food taste better and feelings feel deeper and colors brighter. It amplifies love. Loss can imbue us with such profound gratitude for what we have, and I will always marvel that the void of death can be what makes us feel most alive.

Marko's three-person funeral is the first and last climbing service I attend. I'll wonder if I owe apologies to the living and the dead. I will be haunted by all the things I never said. To their families. To their friends. To them. I think that feeling is probably ubiquitous no matter how much black we wear. I will be afraid to confront any death even as I continue to chase my own.

15

The only thing you can photograph is light

reflecting off something.

—Garry Winogrand

A string of blue smoke rises from the roof of a small shack and a skinny wind turbine made from scrap metal rattles on rusty bearings. Across a field, a young Quechua girl is collecting water from a stream, and I hear only my footsteps and smell fresh donkey shit as a pile smears underfoot. I like the organic scent the way I like the smell of my own sweat because it's real. The girl turns toward me and I see in a glance that she is sweet without knowing. I turn off the trail toward her as she hops through the wet meadow the same way I do, and we speak the same language for a moment. "Hola . . ." I wave and smile and she smiles back but doesn't reply because she's shy. I use my best broken Spanish to ask if I may make a picture of her. She doesn't understand, so I motion at my camera like I have so many times, asking permission through a rough game of charades. It's a universal language like nodding or winking. I wink and she nods and holds the jug at her side.

She fidgets as I squat and compose. Her eyes dart up and down the trail and I think she's a little worried that her chores are being interrupted and doesn't want anyone to see. It's late in the day and dinner needs to be made and hands and feet need to be washed and pans cleaned and dried. But she gives me the time and I take pictures as she looks left and right and behind her. But there is no one in sight. She turns and stares past the camera because she is taking a picture of me too, and for maybe the fourth time in my life, I feel an image as it's made.

I say "Gracias" in a hushed tone because I'm embarrassed by my accent and she answers, "Regalo mi?" which means "My gift?" I make a gesture like I forgot and then hold out a handful of Jolly Ranchers and say, "Dos." She picks *tres*, two watermelons and an apple, which are my favorite flavors too. She smiles and I wink. I think she'd rather have some money, but I have none and sugar is a fabulous runner-up. She hurries ahead toward the wind turbine, which is spinning furiously and making a little hum. I wave but she doesn't see, out of my world just as fast as she crashed in, not knowing just how much her face will change my life. The whole interaction lasts two minutes. I keep walking and smell the donkey shit.

I forget about the picture for two months until I dust it off on a flight from Lima to Houston. I don't sleep because I never can when I'm this tired. The flight attendant offers me a cheap snack bag of dry pretzels in a whisper. I open it quietly and hope the crunch of my jaws won't wake the snoring men on either side of me as I wonder at the parallel pursuits of climbing and photography.

Some of the climbing pictures are good. Some of the pictures from the markets and towns and dark bars are okay. There is a picture of a woman running across an empty street, her body disconnected from her shadow like Peter Pan, and I think it's a little piece of magic.

An hour passes before the portrait of the girl crosses the screen and I stare, noticing the details I was too busy to see before. It's emotional and a world apart from all the other thousands of pictures. She's wearing a stretched pink turtleneck under a pilled, threadbare gray fleece. Her cheeks are dirty and wind-chapped and wisps of backlit hair frame perfectly symmetrical, almond eyes. The expression is timid but connected, and I zoom in. The whites of her eyes are too white, the corners are packed with dirt and crust, and the irises and pupils are completely obscured by a sharp reflection of me. I've taken a self-portrait of someone else's face. The picture has as much to do with me as her and we are locked in a moment that belongs to both of us. I wonder what she was seeing and what the world looks like to her.

Photography, and especially photojournalism, is paradoxical. We imagine photographs as reliable purveyors of truth, but they are all subjective representations. Pieces of truth. "Objectivity" is an unreachable concept because we come to any circumstance carrying our own baggage. The idea that we can tell stories uninfluenced by our own emotional universe is fiction. Even the most journalistic images are their own little deceits. That doesn't mean that they aren't true. It just hints at the fundamental unease of photography: to remove ourselves completely from a photo means that it ceases to exist. I will always be in the picture. If we look hard enough at anything, we can see ourselves reflected back.

The girl's portrait is a quantum leap in my photography and I see years into my future. This image is what I want from art. For now, it's just a glimpse, not an evolution. It's a point on a map, but there is a vast distance between where I am and where I want to be and no clear path between. Instead, I will follow a trail of images as breadcrumbs. A monastery. A flood plain. A cave. Avalanche debris. A blurry bedroom. They will happen one by one and I'll never really know when or where the next will appear.

Over my career, I'll be asked thousands of times what comes first: photography or exploration? It's a lazy question. For me, exploration is a pathway to the hidden lives of others, whether they are the people I stumble across or climb with. Adventure is useful insofar as it brings me closer to stories that are inaccessible to others. The moments collected are just attempts to connect in a disconnected world. I'll eventually learn that I don't need adventure for that. I'll learn that I never wanted to be an adventure photographer. In time, I'll understand that photography and exploration can't be separated because they are the same thing. I look again at the screen. A girl stares at me in a field and I stare back, the two of us entangled as reflections of each other.

I sit back and brush crumbs from my belly and drink the last sip of watered-down ginger ale and smell airplane farts. Eventually I start snoring too. Two hours later I'm woken by the screech of touchdown and look at my ticket to remind me where I am.

16

Leave me to my own absurdity.

—SOPHOCLES

nes Papert scrapes at dark granite above while little pieces of snow fall on me. I pull up my hood and squeeze my eyes, bowing my head and tucking the lower half of my face into my collar. I shake from the cold and can smell my foul breath, which is the only warm piece of me.

Ines breathes heavily and does what she does best, connecting tiny features on blank rock in a way that no one else can. She is arguably the best all-around female climber in the world, equally talented in all disciplines of climbing. Mixed climbing, when you use your ice axes to move between rock and ice seamlessly, is what Ines is famous for. Good climbers make this look like a loud, scratchy battle and they scrape and crawl and shake. Great climbers make it look like a quiet dance and move in a smooth, fluid motion. Ines is a great climber, and I'm in love with her.

The Khumbu Valley below is deep and folded, sculpted by the Dudh Kosi River as it rushes from the glaciers to the jungle and rice paddies below. A maze of boulders and long walls of stone plates carved with Tibetan mantras lead through villages and teahouses with yaks tied and snorting outside. The valley bottom smells of pine and rhododendron and burning juniper. Prayer flags flutter in colorful strips from Buddhist shrines and monasteries, and you can hear chanting monks and bells and smell candle wax coming from the large red doors. One monastery claims to have a piece of a yeti skull, which is probably a black bear, but it's more fun to believe. There are danfe birds colored like peacocks and musk deer with sharp fangs and snow leopards that no one sees because most visitors that come to this place are only looking for one thing: Everest. Or, as it's known here, Chomolungma.

In the spring and fall, the valley is choked with tourists who rely on the hard labor of porters and Sherpas, which are not the same thing. Sherpas are a distinct Tibetan ethnic group and do most of the high-altitude heavy lifting of Himalayan climbing and without them most mountains would never get climbed at all. Porters are usually the heavy lifters of the valley bottoms, shuttling goods and supplies up and down the trails. Their legs are sinewy and strong and they often wear sandals to 17,000 feet. From behind, they look like overfilled baskets with legs because they don't carry backpacks. They call the baskets *dokos* and carry them with a broad strap across their forehead. When they're tired they sit on short, T-shaped walking sticks called *takmos*. But it's winter now and the valley is quiet and empty, leaving Ines and me to make slow progress up a big, empty mountain face.

It's our fifth night on the wall, and we've dug a snow cave big enough for one and a half people and are spooning with our sleeping bags zipped together. I've come a long way from sleeping on ledges with Dad and I stare out of the snow hole and look for Ursa Minor but can't find it. Ines is sleeping and I'm a little scared because the snow below is not solid.

I hear a crack but can't do anything before the bottom collapses and we're falling in a tangled mess, careening over 3,000 feet of stone before we hit the bottom, still tied together.

Ines sleeps and I know I would never be here without her. She is the bold one and takes all the hard sections of the climb while I lead the easier snow and ice fields. My job is to take pictures and film as often as I can when my hands aren't too cold or shaking too much. I tuck my head under the sleeping bag and scroll through the climb and think again that I want more from photography. Climbing is beautiful, but it feels incomplete.

Ines rolls and I turn the camera off and whisper, "I love you."

"I love you too," she says. But I know she doesn't. And maybe I love the idea of her rather than who she really is. Probably. Definitely. I want to be a part of her world and absorb her talents. I hope that osmosis is real.

It's morning now and we crawl off the north face and feel the first sun in six days. Ines is balancing up a blank granite slab and I can't understand what the points of her crampons are standing on because from here it looks like glass. I'm in awe of her and think she's beautiful despite chapped lips that scratch when she kisses me. Because of them. She moves quietly and I love that my hands are no longer cold and I can feel my fingers and toes.

The rope is in one hand and I take pictures and film with the other. Despite the risk, pictures are my contribution here and I yell encouragements after her, hoping she doesn't fall and rip the cord from my hand. She says nothing and it's silent aside from metal on rock and breath and the rustle of nylon clothes.

She's scratching for a crack or ledge or some tiny crystal with her ice axe when her foot skates off, leaving her off-balance on unstable holds. I drop the camera and reach for the rope as her body swings outward like a barn door. But just as it seems there is no way to recover, her ice axe catches a solid hold. Her foot comes back to the rock. She inhales, pulls, scrambles two more easy moves, stands, and screams. From here it's an easy hour to the summit and I know we've just done something significant in the climbing world.

An hour later we're on top and I'm taking pictures of the valley and the mountains and the dark cirque we've just climbed out of. My brain is on fire and I want more of it all. My brain is greedy. I want more *from* it all.

Back in base camp two days later, I'm feeling curious and go for a walk down the valley and turn onto a faint, unmarked trail that I assume leads to nowhere. I climb a steep hillside and hear a bell and see an animal that's half cow and half yak, called a *dzomo* (pronounced like zo-key-o). There are other, English words for this animal that I will learn, like *yattle* and *yakow* and my favorite, *cak*. A tiny structure with a dirt roof is cut into a small terrace in the trees. Left of it is a deep-red wall with one window and a heavy wooden door. The tiny cave monastery is built under the eave of a boulder, and I see a handsome man who speaks no English wave and I say, "Namaskarā, tashi delek." Hello. He runs inside the hermitage and returns with a tin cup, its enamel chipped, filled with hot tea and bits of dirt floating on top, and says, "Chai." I understand because tea is the universal language of the Himalaya.

I don't know if he's a monk or caretaker, but it really doesn't matter because he's here and I'm here and he seems happy to have company. I motion toward the locked door to the cave and point to my eyes and he nods enthusiastically because he's proud of wherever we are.

He fumbles with the lock as the cak shakes its bell and we bend to step inside. The room is 15 feet square and the ceiling is stone. It's dark and smells like incense and the dirt floor holds a hint of mold. Small wooden platforms with Tibetan rugs line the walls, and I ask, "How old?" But he misunderstands and rocks his hand from side to side to say "about" and then holds up seven fingers and then makes the shape of a zero. He's about seventy but isn't really keeping track. I say, "No . . . this," and gesture to the room. He laughs and scrunches his lips and looks to the ceiling as if he is thinking. He rocks his hand again more slowly and shrugs and gives up and says, "Old."

My eyes adjust and the walls come alive, painted with muted frescoes of Buddhist deities sitting on lotus flowers and mandalas and blue monsters with fangs that dance on flaming skulls, and he says "Buddha, Buddha," to make sure I know who's in charge here.

I motion to my camera and point to him, the way I've learned, and he says, "Chitō." Quickly. He has many things to do. There is a yakow to milk and feed. There is firewood to collect and *dal bhat* to heat and rice to cook. There is much tea to drink and scriptures to read and a string of beads to pass endlessly between forefinger and thumb. Most importantly, there is silence to sit in. Even in solitude, there is much to do.

He looks for the stool behind him as he sits down and stares at my camera and I learn one of the most important lessons of photography: some of the best portraits take the least amount of time. Sometimes the first glance is the most honest moment before they start pretending. Other times you have to exhaust someone before they show you something real.

After a minute we agree we're done and step outside as he locks the door behind us. The overcast day seems brighter now and the yattle rings its bell because it is time to go. The trail back down is steep, and the man calls after me, "Bistārī, bistārī," slowly, slowly, and waves.

Back in base camp I hunch over my screen in an oversized down jacket because I'm never warm here. The portrait of the man's face is evenly lit, and his eyes are gently overhung with aging skin. There is a ring of light in his pupils from the flash and the background is deep black. His cheekbones are fleshy and hang as if his face is slowly being pulled back to the earth and reclaimed.

A day later news has broken in the climbing world. This website says, "Ines Papert debuts in the Himalaya with Cory Richards and forges 'Cobra Norte' up the North Face of Kwangde Shar 6093m, Nepal, Himalaya," and that website says, "Huge new line established in the Khumbu." Editors request pictures of the face and I draw a red line showing our climb winding its way from feature to feature like a cobra and insert little yellow triangles to show where we slept. Ines emails all the images to her sponsors. She is traversing an ice field. She's in a snow cave. She's inching her way up a blank slab and the sun is a hot-white star. This is her success more than mine. I know it. She knows it. Everyone knows it. But I don't mind. I don't need to be the best, so long as I'm in the game.

In one image, Ines is rounding the corner of the face onto the summit ridge. Beyond her, I can see the mountains of Dad's books stepping back in fading layers. There is Makalu, the fifth-highest mountain, and there is Lhotse, the fourth-highest. There is Tawoche and Cholatse and Ama Dablam. There is the enormous wall called Nuptse, which guards the highest of them all, Everest.

I'm addicted and stare at all the tiny dots on the map of my future. Over the next two years I will fail on Makalu twice. I'll climb Lhotse, fail on Nupste twice, and summit Ama Dablam. Next winter I'll climb a new route on Tawoche with Renan Ozturk and we'll post episodic dispatches from high on the mountain, huddling above our computers while our faces glow blue above cold hands. In doing so, we'll help usher in a new era of real-time storytelling long before Instagram and Snapchat and TikTok.

Every climb bleeds into the next in dizzying succession until I'm spending more time in Nepal than home.

It's May 2010 and Conrad Anker and I are standing in Everest base camp watching an avalanche. I call him "Rad" or "Radish" or "Deesh" and admire him fiercely. He deserves most of the credit for my climbing career but on this day he opens a far bigger door when he forwards an email from *National Geographic* photo editor Susan Welchman, who's asking for pictures of the effort to remove trash from Everest.

I take an image of a porter standing ankle-deep in garbage throwing heaps of shit over the camera, and I beg a neighboring camp to use their satellite internet to email it back to D.C. Susan's words are encouraging but she's not satisfied: "It's good, but I need something more. I need something unexpected."

Two days later, I hear that a mummified hand is melting from the ice. It's white and wrinkled like it's been underwater too long but I can still see the fingerprints and I wonder who it was while I take pictures. Susan says, "This is working. But I need more."

I don't know what can top a mummified hand until someone tells me they recovered a watch from the wrist. The strap is frayed and creased and the face has no glass. On the back is a small, cursive inscription of someone's initials: J.C.R. I think of their last moments and the name the initials stand for. I wonder when time ended for them and kept going for everyone else. The rusted hands read 1:05.

I photograph the fragments on a sheet of white paper and Susan says, "*Yes!* This is perfect! Thank you for your work!"

"You're welcome! I hope to work with you again."

"Me too. It's like dancing with a good partner."

Seven months later, three of my images are published in the most widely recognized magazine in the world and I look at my name printed next to them in small, neat letters. It's a start.

I know the best climbers are usually quiet and out beyond cameras, often dodging the attention of media. I know I'm not the most talented, but I'm talented enough. I have a talent for relentlessness to the point of annoyance. A talent for being a bit crazy and a bit brazen and a bit stupid. A talent for telling stories. A talent for being loved and loathed. Talented enough behind the camera and delighted to be in front of it. I'm talented at wearing many hats and faces and jackets and all of them are distinct but overlapping versions of me.

Over three years I go to the Himalaya twelve times and make thousands of images and an artistic evolution is clear. A cohesive voice is emerging, and it's mine.

The backgrounds stretch back hundreds of miles into the highest, most inaccessible mountains in the world. A small person climbs above an impossible landscape in a red jacket, dwarfed by glaciers that bend and wind and crack. Now I'm above the clouds and the world is glowing pink. Now a tent is perched on a ledge that falls away into nothing. All of them are beautiful and I love turning a page and finding an image of something so big, something that bends the imagination. These pictures answer questions of possibility and potential and capacity. They inspire.

But for every ten thousand images of the extraordinary, the ones that stop me are the quiet, hidden moments. It's the thousand-yard stare of exhaustion. A man in prayer. A hermit in a dark room. A mummified hand and a watch. Interesting pictures always ask more questions than they answer.

I take other pictures too and they are of the shadows made by all the bright light of my growing success. They are faceless and the things no one shows. A nameless lover in a hotel room as she sits in a window with a cigarette and her robe falls open. A blurry image while we have sex. Sometimes they are of dark places that only I know. Dirty sheets and a handprint on the green wall of a brothel. A stripper's fake eyelashes on a windowsill next to an empty bottle. A friend bent over a rolled-up dollar bill and a chalky mirror. Still-lifes of my mind and many secrets.

More than my mountain pictures, I return to these other images again and again and again and wonder why the imperfect instants of blur and rough edges always say so much. These intimate, fragile moments are an expression of my deepest, most honest voice. I know why the quiet frames of empty rooms scream. I'm haunted by what I hide and scared that if I show the world everything, I'll be erased.

Photography is just light reflecting off the world around us. Even my most technically "perfect" pictures will always be referred to as "raw" and I'll hate this until I understand it. It's the intangible emotional transaction between photographer, subject, and viewer that makes pictures powerful and now I'm thinking of the way the little girl stared at me in the field in Peru and I wonder again what she might have seen. Maybe she saw it all. Or maybe she was just a child fetching water.

What I can see is that all pictures are connected in some fundamental way. The girl is the hermit and he is the man in the tent who is the person in prayer who is the lover in the open robe. She is the handprint on the wall that holds the dollar bill. I don't understand their lives but I know that we share more than we don't, even our secrets. I am them and we are me, separated by oceans and years and experience and privilege and language. We are all overlapping stories woven together like a tapestry that blankets the world and that is what all the light is reflecting off of. We are a daisy chain of eight billion reflections.

I'm twenty-nine. My childhood memories feel like someone else's, sharp but distant. The world sees me, a piece of me at least, and my star is rising.

I was twenty-one when my first image was published. The eight years since have produced hundreds of publications and thousands of miles and hundreds of thousands of pictures, condensing as much experience as I could to build my little mountain of success. I've built a reputation as an able climber and an ambitious storyteller and now I'm on the phone and hear a high-pitched Italian voice say, "So, we leave December 27." I hang up and call Dad, who says, "Go gently," and I say, "I'll call you from Islamabad."

17

إِنْ شَاءَ ٱللَّهُ [if God wills].

—ARABIC PROVERB

'm eight and Dad is next to me on the chairlift. It's clear and cold with rays of sun splitting snow crystals that seem to float up as much as down. Dad isn't wearing gloves because he never does, no matter how cold it is, and his hands look big to me. But my hands are frozen, so he removes my gloves one at a time and blows three hot breaths in each. I love how warm they are when I put them back on but hate how his breath makes them feel a little wet inside. His patrol radio crackles and says something I don't understand and Dad looks at me and says, "Watch this," pointing toward the mountain above.

There is a pop from somewhere and then a boom, and a tiny puff of black smoke rises from the top of a big chute. The snow splinters and collapses into a fractal web and begins to slide. Seconds later, the avalanche explodes out of the bottom of the chute like a huge boiling cloud.

"Would that kill someone?" I ask. I'm fascinated and have no sense of scale.

"Every time," Dad answers without looking away. I love avalanches but understand that they demand respect and fear.

Mom speaks French and teaches me that *avalanche* is a word from the seventeenth century and came from another Old French word, *avaler,* which means "to descend." That became the modern verb that means "to swallow." But Dad says that in the mountains the definition of *avalanche* is "oh fuck" and I love when he swears.

Dad teaches me that a slab avalanche happens when wind redeposits ice crystals on a slope, creating a dense layer of compacted snow that gets heavier and heavier. Billions of once unrelated particles are patiently deposited to form a singular, bound structure. Crystal by crystal, the density and weight of the slab increase, waiting to descend and swallow everything below. It's an equation of time and pressure.

Anything can trigger an avalanche. The weight of a bird. A minuscule rise in temperature. A climber's foot. Just the wind. Eventually gravity takes over and the weak layers of snow underneath the slab collapse. The slope splinters into an enormous, inescapable spiderweb.

The web becomes a mass of snow, ice, and rock that can move as fast as 200 feet per second. Large avalanches can create an air blast that pushes out in front of them, snapping full-grown trees like matchsticks. In 1945, the air blast of Hiroshima exerted 16 kilotons of force. Massive avalanches can impact with 7.6 kilotons, just under half the power of an atomic bomb.

I look at Dad and ask, "What do you do if you get caught?" The plume has cleared and the mountain seems eerily silent.

"All you can. Swim like hell. Pray." He looks at me and smiles. "Better yet, just don't get caught."

I sit with Simone Moro and Denis Urubko in the cold dining room of a guesthouse in Islamabad, Pakistan, and huddle in my down jacket wondering how we will ever climb a mountain in this season. It's December 28, 2010. We're tired and jetlagged and still waking up. The walls are white. Or blue. But I'll always remember all of it as gray. Gray clouds. Gray streets. Gray buildings. Gray tasks. December is a dismal month in Islamabad. The sun seems tired and lazy and barely breaks through the wet mist before giving up for the day.

I'm picking the skin off the top of my coffee and remember meeting Simone and Denis on my first trip to the Himalaya with Ines, the same season they did the first winter ascent of Makalu, the world's fifth-highest mountain. Simone and I became friends a year later at Everest base camp while he attempted to climb the mountain without oxygen. I climbed Lhotse and sang an off-key rendition of Céline Dion's "All by Myself" as I sat alone at 8,516 meters, or 27,940 feet. But I feel out of place now and understand my value is more as a camera than as a climber.

Over the next four days we attend a blur of meetings with the military and various ministries and officials. Shopping and packing and repacking because the tension must escape somehow. A cup of tea. A cup of coffee. A hidden drink of whiskey shared in secret because alcohol is against the law. Permits and a feast of mutton and chicken and more tea. I take pictures and film everything because this is my job, but also because I want to justify my presence. Even though I know Simone, I'm an outsider in his well-established dynamic with Denis, who makes no effort to hide his reservations about me and says, "But Simone, it is maybe not possible for Cory." I feel like an imposter and wonder if he's right.

Denis's eyes are very blue and match his jacket and I think he's small for a Himalayan mountaineering giant, just slightly bigger than me. He has thin, short brown hair that lays flat and grows from a high widow's peak framing defined cheekbones and a thin face. The bridge of his nose is broader than the tip and he reminds me of a villain. He speaks with a thick Russian accent that drops words, replaces nouns with verbs, exchanges *w* and *v,* and mixes tenses, and he is always singing "Volare." This undermines his Russian severity, which will eventually dissolve altogether into an enduring brotherhood. But that will take being tied together for six exhausting weeks. I don't yet know that he lived under bridges and fought his way up from the streets. I don't know that climbing saved his life in much the same way it has mine and that he chose to risk his life in order to save it. He's climbed all fourteen 8,000-meter peaks without oxygen. Death is better than the world he's risen from.

Simone's eyes are dark with heavy lids, hidden behind glasses. He is mousy and chiseled with a sideways smile and slightly crooked teeth. His voice is a high-pitched rasp so distinct that I would recognize it in the loudest room. When he starts telling me about beautiful bitches, I squirm. "Cory, you must come to see the Italian bitches! Most beautiful bitches in the world!" It will be days before I realize he hasn't learned English from American hip-hop but is inviting me to see Italy's stunning coastline. Beautiful beaches. If we survive, I will come to see the bee-ches.

The day after I agree to a seaside vacation, we crawl into an enormous helicopter called an MI-17 that looks more like a tank with a propeller on top. A crew of five Pakistani Army officers wearing knock-off Oakley sunglasses and green aviator headphones maneuvers the flying dinosaur over the great, braided basin of the Shigar and Braldu Rivers. Black and blue and green water snakes its way around thousands of islands of gray stone, carving grooves through the old seabed like the sinewy tail of a horse. The foothills grow into the granite teeth of the Karakorum and the helicopter whines and purrs and shakes against air that I know must be too thin to support the weight of eight men and thousands of pounds of gear. My mouth dries up and I drink water so I can swallow, and I hide my panic by smiling awkwardly at Denis and Simone. The noise of the engine is too loud to speak over, so I motion and nod and make faces of awe and hope that they can't see my fear.

The river below disappears into the broad tongue of the Baltoro Glacier. Sharp orange spires rise to my left. These are the Trango Towers, some of the most storied mountains in the world. Just as quickly as they rise, they suddenly seem small in comparison to the mountains around them.

Thirty minutes later the glacier is a mile wide with ribbons of white snow and black stone. There is K2, the second-highest mountain in the world, rising as an impossible black pyramid with a tail of white blowing from its summit. The helicopter turns right and I crane my neck up the icy slopes of Broad Peak, the twelfth-highest. Ten minutes later the pitch of the engine changes and the motion slows. The Godwin-Austen Glacier below us is pure white and protests the rotors with billows of icy dust. I think of the snow crystals floating upward as I sat next to Dad.

The first thing I notice is the carcass of an identical helicopter, crashed and frozen in the ice. The second thing I notice is how dry and cold the air is. When I inhale, my nostrils freeze closed. In ten minutes, my toes are tiny stumps that I have to warm over a stove before finding my mountaineering boots, which are buried in one of the thirty duffels that the helicopter dumped before flying off and leaving us in a great white silence.

For the first time I stare up at the thirteenth-highest point on the planet, Gasherbrum II, the mountain we've come to climb. My heart sinks because it's too big and too high and too much and for the first time I ask myself, "What the fuck am I doing here?"

A Pakistani soldier with a big beard and stained teeth smokes a Marlboro Red and looks at me confused before smiling and saying, "As-salamu alaykum." Peace be upon you. He nods toward the mountain and says, "Climbing?"

I smile and reply, "We try."

"In sha'Allah." If God wills. He exhales and walks away, disappearing into a structure that appears to be made entirely of discarded jerry cans frozen together in a heap.

Tonight we sleep in a fiberglass igloo, one of twenty or so tiny structures that the Pakistani Army inhabits 365 days a year. The outside is white, made to blend into the landscape the soldiers are defending from India. But the real enemy here isn't bullets or a foreign flag. It's crevasses and altitude and avalanches. It's cold and exposure and boredom. It's the cancer from the cigarettes and diabetes from the endless cups of milky chai. Like avalanches themselves, the enemy here is time and pressure.

Within weeks, we settle into a familiar rhythm of climbing higher and higher on the mountain and I watch Simone and Denis stumble through crevasses and up ice slopes. I hold my breath as we sneak under enormous hanging ice cliffs that break off and fall in thunderous avalanches, washing away our tracks. We place small bamboo wands along our path to mark the way and tell us where cracks in the ice are hiding and leave piles of gear buried in the snow. Climb high, sleep low. Climb higher. Sleep higher. Go back to base camp. Rest. Repeat as our bodies build red blood cells that carry oxygen and allow us, maybe, to climb all the way to the top.

Two weeks later I squint down from a rib of ice thousands of feet above base camp. But the colorful tents are too far away to see, hidden beneath the yawning glacial valley under my feet. A broken superhighway of ice and snow appears as a maze of crevasses that separates us from the safety of the kerosene and tea and movies I saved on my laptop. I look up but can't see the mountain I'm here to climb because I'm on it. I've lost the forest through the trees and my breath is a rhythmic tether that calms my mind when it all seems too big. And it always seems too big.

Every morning I take the same pink and purple pills that keep me sane. Valproic acid and bupropion. One pill to temper my volatility and keep the racing thoughts at bay. One to make me happy. By now I've taken them for fifteen years and wonder if they do anything at all. But I don't wonder anymore at the irony of staying sane to do insane things to escape insanity. In some way I know that they all rely on each other. The only places where I feel normal are where nothing is normal at all.

The cold no longer registers because my body has adjusted, and instead of paying attention to the pain in my fingers and toes I watch as pieces of ice fall between my boots and bounce 1,000 feet before disappearing. It's not that I'm not cold—I am. But the only way to get warmer is to move, so I keep moving. Kick the spikes of my crampons into the blue ice, step up. Swing the pick of my ice axe, pull up. Breathe and kick. Step and swing. Pull and breathe. Every motion is an act of defiance against my better sense.

The avalanches that pour off the mountains are now just background percussion to the more delicate notes of my immediate surroundings and the lyrics that get stuck in my head. The Smashing Pumpkins loop in my mind, "And we don't know just where our bones will rest / To dust, I guess, forgotten and absorbed into the earth below."

The thin air makes the noises of our movement so clear it startles me and I look over my shoulder in search of the person that made them. But it's just me. The lack of atmosphere makes everything appear in sharp focus. Living at high altitude is like living in hi-def. The clarity is unsettling, like watching an awkward love scene in 4K when the pores are too sharp and the kissing too loud. In moments, I long for the muted existence of home.

On days when it's too cold or stormy or when we need to rest, I wander over to the Pakistani Army post next to base camp and spend hours with the soldiers, drinking tea until I'm jittery from the caffeine and sugar and my teeth hurt. Some speak excellent English and some none, but it doesn't matter because we are all fascinated by each other. We're nothing like we expected each other to be but seem unable to understand what those expectations were to begin with.

Their village of fiberglass igloos is connected by dirty trails of packed snow. The interiors are dark with a few round windows to let out the smoke that blackens the walls with soot. There is a small sea of stained, military-green down sleeping bags that smell like unwashed bodies and cigarettes and kerosene stoves. I can't read the Arabic scribbles of names, inside jokes, and verses from the Koran scratched into the blackness. Next to them are hashmarks of hours and months and I understand them immediately. These are the universal language of time passing too slowly.

Sometimes I watch *Terminator* or *Platoon* or *Apocalypse Now* with the soldiers. Their favorites are Rambo films and they jostle each other while repeating, "Live for nothing or die for something!" as a chorus and laugh. Someone makes tea and the light is gorgeous through the steam and smoke. I take a picture.

One night I wander down a small ice ravine near base camp and find a soldier's boot in the ice with a leg bone frozen inside. I take a picture and walk away and wonder who that person was and where the foot had been before it ended up just there.

The soldiers use my computer to check Facebook and I accept all the friend requests from Faizan and Mohammed and Ahmad and wonder if this will put me on the TSA watch list. Some days we sit in silence and stare at the stoves and sip tea while they feed me fresh chapatis with spicy pickles called achar. I'm not one of them but they treat me as such and it feels sweet. I can't tell if it's pride, humor, or duty when they say, "Well, back to being a martyr!" as they bundle up and walk back into the cold. It seems like this is a phrase they all know. I take another picture.

A detail returns from a forward operating post on Conway Saddle, which is the highest territory Pakistan holds in its conflict with India. The soldiers look tired and thin. Their cheeks and lips are cracked, and their beards are full and unkempt. The younger soldiers seem to fall more than walk because they've been living just below 20,000 feet for weeks. An officer who's just arrived from below stands in his spotless white uniform next to another who is returning from the high ground. His suit is dark gray and stained from the same kerosene smoke that makes the igloos black and I wonder what this is doing to their lungs. One is excited because he doesn't know anything. The other is relieved to never know again. I take a picture.

I watch a soldier hang a purple tracksuit on a clothesline and it freezes instantly into a stiff pancake. A small, sun-bleached Pakistani flag with little unraveled fibers waves above an igloo. The skeleton of the crashed helicopter says "Army" on the tail and casts a distorted shadow on the snow and seems like a joke about war, but no one is laughing. I take pictures of all of it.

After four weeks nothing seems new and I marvel at how quickly unfamiliar experiences transform into mundane reality. The cold is just cold. The wind is just wind. I take photos without my gloves even though the thermometer says −33 and I think of Dad. I coax my laptop back to life every morning with a thermos of hot water against the battery and string out short film dis-

patches just like I learned from Renan, uploading them to a production house in Europe so people can follow along on our grand
adventure. I hide in my tent at base camp and watch *Spy Game*
for the sixty-third time and imagine what it would be like to
have a job where dying is a real possibility until I realize I do. I
listen to Mitch Hedberg tell jokes about going to base camp just
so he can grow a beard and drink hot chocolate and the punch
line comes: "'You goin' to the top?' . . . 'Soon.'"

I fall asleep to jokes I've heard hundreds of times because they
are reliable and comfortable.

Hermann Hesse's *Siddhartha* sits in the mesh pocket of my base
camp tent. Twenty-nine days ago I grabbed it from the shelf just
before my new fiancée, Liv, drove me to the airport. I asked if I
could borrow it and was surprised when she didn't say yes immediately. Instead, she pulled it from my hand, opened it briefly
like she was looking for something, and handed it back. "Sure,
baby, just bring it home." I noticed the gold ring that I put on her
finger two days earlier when I asked her to marry me in a restaurant that neither of us really liked and I felt guilty for not trying
harder. At the very least I could've chosen a better restaurant and
drunk less wine. But I knew the answer would be yes before I
asked, so I was lazy. I also knew I shouldn't have asked and some
nights I fall asleep trying to love her more.

I think of her when I open the book two days before we leave
for the summit push. I think of love and wonder if this is what
everyone talks about. Inside the book is an inscription in a man's
handwriting I don't recognize. It says:

Liv,
    Timing is everything.
                                    Love, Nick

Nick was her former love. But Nick died in an avalanche. His words will haunt me.

The night before we leave, Simone takes a call from a Swiss man named Karl Gabl and talks in his high-pitched Italian accent while I film. The thermometer says –26 while the wind whips at the nylon walls of the cook tent and the day fades from white to black. I notice the condensation of the stoves dripping from the walls and freezing in a rim of icicles. Karl says the weather forecast is "marginal but promising." Simone hangs up the phone, removes his glasses, and massages between his eyes. He looks up at Denis and me. "So, tomorrow we go."

I wake up at 7 A.M. and wash down my antidepressants and mood stabilizers with lukewarm water and eat fresh chapatis with honey dyed yellow to make it look like it came from bees. The chai is thick and milky and full of caffeine, which makes me even more anxious, and I step out of the door into overcast skies. It's –15°C and I think it feels warm this morning.

Everything is an act of superstition as I mimic the motions of a thousand previous climbs that didn't kill me. Which glove goes on first? I wear three necklaces. One has an auspicious Buddhist stone that is said to protect its wearer. Another is a pendant of a Norse talisman, Ullr, the patron of snow, who is said to paint the northern lights with the spray from his skis. The third is of a Catholic saint. I'm trying to cover my spiritual bases. I lace up the clunky boots and try to remember which crampon I always put on first.

The day is all storm, wind, and white, interrupted by the three dots of color snaking our way up the icefall and listening to avalanches we can't see. Simone and Denis are unfazed. I jump every time I hear the rumble and scan the mountain for the white haunting and hope the sounds are not the ghosts of some future inevitability.

On the morning of January 31, I pull on a puffy one-piece down suit and feel like an astronaut blasting off into outer space as we crawl from the tent into another overcast day. Above us the pitch steepens. From here it's 2,000 meters of climbing to the top of the near-perfect, light gray summit pyramid covered in a layer of frost.

The first slope sounds hollow beneath us and sends out fractures and great *whoomph*s, signaling that the snow is unstable and ready to avalanche. I try to tiptoe in an arcing traverse to reach the bottom of a long, steep couloir, knowing that there is no way to be lighter on my feet. I don't pray but I make promises and deals with all the gods hanging from my neck because my relationship with the divine is purely transactional.

The wind blows spindrift down the chute and obscures my vision, so I bow my head and feel cold crystals collect around the exposed skin of my neck. My breath and body heat freeze a film across my goggles and I'm annoyed I can't see. The fog makes me claustrophobic and anxious. But I keep climbing and limit words in exchange for breaths that seem too short, like I'm always coming to the surface of water.

I'd be lying if I said there isn't a sense of freedom and joy under the fear. The joy is thin like the air and is never enough, so I breathe deeper and try to hold on to all of it. I love this despite the fear and I love this because of the fear and I hate it for all the same reasons. I remember Andre Agassi again and think I finally understand what he means when he says, "I hate tennis."

After six hours the three of us crawl into a tent made for two and look like big down-filled sardines. I stuff wet socks into my jacket to dry and pull dry socks on over swampy, wrinkled feet. Dad taught me the best way to dry everything is to stuff it into my sleeping bag and let the heat of my body push through the fibers. But nothing is ever really dry here. Instead, everything hovers somewhere between damp and frozen. The inside of the tent becomes a dense fog of unwashed breath, laughter, and

phlegmy coughs that beg for water. I film the scene through
fogged lenses and hope that the condensation doesn't fry the
camera altogether.

On February 1, I lead the team higher on the mountain than
we've been. The sky is deep blue and crisp with stringy wisps of
white called mares' tails, signaling moisture and high wind in the
upper atmosphere. A storm is coming. The mountains behind us
look like rows of teeth, layer upon layer of sharp summits that
appear like the mouth of a shark. When the sun is out and the
wind stops, I understand that there is no place in this world or
any other where I belong more. When it blows, I wish to be anywhere else.

At 6,800 meters we carve a platform in the ice under the overhanging lip of a large crevasse, pitch the sardine can, and eat
Simone's wife's homemade tortellini. Denis sings "Volare" again
in his Russian accent while Simone calls home on the satellite
phone and talks in a baby voice to his infant son. He calls Karl to
check the weather and answers him in German and Italian and
English high above a landscape of Urdu, Pashto, and Balti and
the world seems big and small, and I think of my former life as a
Christian. Genesis 11:1–9. We are camped high on the Tower of
Babel in a world confused by languages, wearing big puffy one-
sies, reaching for some perverse version of heaven. I call my
parents and Mom says, "Good luck, sweetheart. Make smart decisions." I say, "I love you," because this is the language of our
family. Every language says the weather will be clear and stable
for the next eighteen hours. Simone says, "In sha'Allah," and
Denis says, "In sha'Allah!" and I say, "Okay . . ."

We wake just after midnight on February 2 and pull on the frozen outer shells of our boots and drink water that tastes like gas
and metal. Simone coughs more violently and Denis talks to

himself in Russian. The watch hanging from the ceiling is covered in the same thick layer of frost covering everything else. It falls from the ceiling of the tent and tickles my face and neck. I look at the temperature: –51°C. I do the math in my head to check for the mental confusion that signals altitude sickness. That's –60° Fahrenheit, give or take.

We crawl from the tent into a moonless night and look up at a sky that is more stars than space. The air is cold and slams against the back of my throat and makes me cough. I'd murder someone for a cigarette.

The teeth of the shark are a black line against the sky, and our headlamps are the only indication of life for miles. We are tiny, illuminated islands in a sea of snow and stone and I imagine what we look like from above.

My hands are cold and lifeless. I swing them violently in big circles until the blood rushes back in as a searing pain and I don't know if I want to scream or vomit. But this pain is good. It means my limbs are flowing with blood and for now altitude hasn't caught up with my body. The only thing that can make this endeavor safe is speed and today is a race against a storm we know is coming. So I stare at the snow in the glow of my island of light and chase the steam of my own breath as it rises into the night. We are thread and time is a needle.

I've always hated the term "death zone," which refers to elevations above 8,000 meters, where the body is actively dying. It's a term used by the uninitiated, armchair mountaineers and media to imbue a sense of danger to a world they know nothing of. But for the first time I respect it. For the first time I feel the death zone all around me.

At some point before dawn the stars begin to fade and a seamless gradient of blue meets the horizon. I pass a pair of boots frozen in the rocks and my brain is slow, so I think it's garbage from a previous expedition. But then I see the legs. And then I see the waist. And finally, I see the whole lifeless body, wrapped in a discarded tent.

As the sun is just about to rise, I run ahead of Denis and Simone. I turn on the camera and try to adjust the exposure, but the buttons and dials are frozen and I have no time to warm them before the sun tips over the horizon, washing Denis in an orange glow against the deep shadows of the world below. This picture will become one of my most famous but the effort it takes has me bent in half and dry-heaving. After thirty seconds, my fingers are numb and the iris of the lens is freezing open. I tuck it away and keep climbing.

Three hours later, Denis and Simone double over in the wind on the summit ridge while they take the last, labored steps toward climbing infamy. Denis raises his hands on the summit and Simone arrives two minutes later and collapses into a fit of coughing while he hides his face from the wind. I arrive as Denis falls to his knees next to him and throws his arms over the hunched shoulders that shudder and convulse. They look like Skittles. I'd skin a cat for some Skittles.

I can't hear what Denis is saying to Simone over the wind. But I don't need to hear to understand. The snow under my boots squeaks and squeals against the metal and rubber. I am the only American to ever climb an 8,000-meter peak in winter. When I write this a decade later, that will still be true. But now, all I know is that there is no time for celebration. The sky is no longer blue but a powder gray as the leading edge of the storm swallows the summit. The watch hanging from my harness says −61°C and I try to do the math again but can't because my brain is too sluggish. My mind is connecting delayed thoughts like I'm drunk and I'm scared because this is fast becoming a game of minutes. I take a picture with Denis and Simone and say a total of seven words: "Let's get the fuck out of here!"

We reverse our steps across the plateau where I took the picture of Denis at sunrise and the sun has dipped behind the summits, replaced by a violent white glow that makes me squint and age. The rays refract off the millions of snow crystals lifted into the air by the storm. Light reflecting off of things. A million tiny shards blast against my skin and turn it white as if the mountain is trying to freeze me in place, jealous of all the color of life.

Denis removes his frozen goggles to see but it roasts his retinas and freezes his eyelids together. Finally, both Simone and Denis relinquish the lead and I'm in front, descending into a void to search for the tent that we hope hasn't blown away.

I find it just before dusk and we crawl in and feel something that resembles safety. I call Dad and lie about what's happening. But he reads between the lines and hides my predicament from Mom. I hear his words before they leave his lips: "Go gently."

I'm almost asleep when the tent lifts off the ground and I hear the nylon tear and we're tomahawking down 1,700 meters in an exploding heap of down and flesh.

I see it happening over and over again like counting dying sheep until some version of rest holds me between sleep and wakefulness.

In the morning, the wind is gusting at 100 kph and the tent is trying to blow away as it traps air like a balloon. I try to film but the camera is frozen, so I shove it into my pack and borrow Simone's small point-and-shoot and forget to film altogether.

When we reach Camp 1, we feel safe for a moment and joke about the descent while the story of survival swells our egos. But we're cocky too soon.

On the morning of February 4, a meter of fresh snow rests under an oppressive ceiling of clouds while Simone breaks trail underneath a mountain called Gasherbrum V. And then, a piece of ice falls or one too many crystals land or the wind blows just wrong and I hear it before I see it. It sounds like thunder and a freight train and wind all at once. Avalanches are like atoms coming together to form a body, trapping energy in a unified structure until life breaks us into a million pieces.

I try to run, but the snow is waist-deep and too heavy. I take three steps before the air blast lifts my body and I'm weightless.

I slam back into the tongue of the avalanche and hear Dad say, "Swim like hell!" But even if I could move my arms and kick against the force, I don't know which direction to paddle because I have no form, tumbling over and over in an exploding heap of down and nylon. But this isn't my colorful imagination. It's real and it has only two colors. Black and white. Black and white. Over and over and over.

I summon all the force I have left and thrust my hand and head toward what I hope is the sky and hear Simone and Denis and the soldiers and everyone in the world say, "*In sha'Allah . . .*"

But you know this story because we're back where we started. It is the middle, which is the end of the beginning and the start of something new. History will carry forward and become the future the way it always does because everything is just now. When it all stops, I pull the camera from my down suit, point it at my face, and take a picture.

18

Blood is really warm, it's like drinking hot chocolate

but with more screaming.

—RYAN MECUM

In the climbing world, we're famous. Sixteen expeditions over twenty-six years had tried and failed to accomplish what we just did. We are the "first" and I'm the "only" and now it's my face on the cover of magazines. We do radio and TV interviews and people want us to speak and write and send them pictures. I'm flying to Europe and Asia and signing books and posters and it all seems a bit silly for climbing an obscure mountain in winter. I sit with Simone and Denis in packed auditoriums for The North Face and know that without them this never would've happened. I also know that without my pictures and the forthcoming film, this success wouldn't be what it is. I know without the footage and the portrait after the avalanche, the wildfire of the aftermath wouldn't be the same. We aren't equal climbers, but we are equal partners.

Anson Fogel's editing suite is nearly black with padded walls and I notice how sounds are soft and final when there is nothing to bounce off. It's strange how silence seems to press against your eardrums in the absence of sound. Three big screens spread out in front of me while Anson hunches and squints, tapping the keyboard as he moves small clips of footage back and forth across the monitors on a timeline. It looks like a scientific picture of sequenced DNA and the clips are the building blocks of a story.

Anson is mostly bald with a very sharp jaw and light eyes that don't know what color they want to be. His goatee is ginger and he always looks severe, holding eye contact until you look away. I like to smoke cigarettes with him and talk about film and make him laugh so he stops looking so mad. He's angry in the same deep way I am, which makes us relate, and we make fun of ourselves because we are both far too serious and know this but can't help it. Taking a break from editing, we stand on the porch in silence until I say, "God, we are such fucking amazing artists. Probably the best in the world!" and he laughs.

"You ready?" he asks as we sit back down in the editing suite.

"Punch it, Chewie."

He taps the space bar and the screens go black. Wind moans as blurry white words fade in:

February 2
21,959 ft.
−51°F

The sound of nylon flapping and whipping in the wind is sharp and the interior of a tent appears, covered in frost. A blurry man in a yellow down suit says something in Russian as the camera focuses on particles of moisture in the steam. Cut to the lens pointing at me. I narrate and the voice in my head says, "What the fuck am I doing here? We have to get down." Cut. Every surface is covered in crystals as the camera pans and it's quiet until a man in red coughs hoarsely. Cut. Snow blows across a shallow icescape and the mournful guitar of Gustavo Santaolalla creeps in, the screen fades to black, and the title, *COLD*, slowly appears and then blows away. It all feels very dramatic and I like the brevity of the name because I always have too many words.

We've been working on the film about Gasherbrum II for months. Anson and I take notes on the audio and timing. I will never like the movie and always see the holes and imperfections, wishing I had filmed more. But many people will love it and it will win awards and people will call it "raw," which I'll still hear as "not very good." *COLD* will carry the story outside of the adventure world and will eventually land on the desk of Chris Johns, the chief editor of *National Geographic*. My portrait will be printed on the cover of the magazine's 125th-anniversary issue and the story will keep living and breathing.

My fiancée, Liv, and I have an old house with a hardwood floor that booms under my feet and is nearly silent under hers. Our kitchen is small and lived in. The cupboards squeak on tired hinges and too many layers of paint make them hard to open and close and the light is a bit too yellow. I'm pacing back and forth talking to a photo editor at *National Geographic* named Sadie Quarrier, wondering what she will say.

Even though I've shot a couple of single-page stories for the magazine, in order to hire me for feature assignments, they need evidence of my ability to shoot an entire, long-form story. They need proof that I understand how to carry a narrative arc through a collection of pictures. When Sadie reached out and asked what I had as an example, I sent her the images from my time with the soldiers in base camp, hoping that it would be enough. No other collection of pictures I have even comes close to what she needs to see.

Liv moves around me silently to grab a teacup. She pours me a glass of wine, kisses me on the cheek, crosses her fingers to say "Good luck," and walks out of the room.

I open and close cabinets and drawers looking for nothing and feel the thick paint stick and listen and fidget as Sadie says, "I love the interiors of these igloos." I'm back on the glacier in Pakistan in a dark dome filled with smoke. I can hear her fingers tapping a keyboard as she scrolls through more images. "I love the purple tracksuit!"

I laugh. "If you gotta go to war, at least go with style."

She tells me she'll call next Tuesday. It's Thursday now, and I count the number of days on my fingers. Four seems like an impossible wait. I know if this door doesn't open now, it probably never will.

Tuesday comes and she sounds disappointed. I know the pictures weren't good enough as she tells me, "I'm so sorry, Cory . . ." while I think of what I can say to convince her. But she continues, "I'm sorry because I'm going to have to ask you to get on a plane and fly to Washington, D.C. We'd like to send you on assignment to Nepal." Six weeks later, I'm blowing sand off my lens.

The Kingdom of Mustang in northern Nepal is a world apart and full of secrets. The Kali Gandaki River funnels off the Tibetan Plateau and carves its way through the center of the sovereignty, flowing through the bottom of a rough gorge that reminds me of the Grand Canyon. It's red and orange and yellow. It's purple and gray. Depending on the season, it's spotted with green terraces and orchards. Unlike the more traveled valleys of the Himalaya, Mustang feels unpolished. It's ancient and always smells like burning yak dung and horseshit and sometimes marijuana, which grows wild in the pastures. Steep canyons with names like the Valley of One Hundred Blind Horses and One Hundred Blind Dogs empty into terraces above the main river bottom, which is braided and wide but seems small beneath the cliffs.

The wind from the Himalaya siphons off the highlands and

funnels through the canyon, whipping up dust storms that sting my cheeks and make me squint. The landscape is parched and burns my face with wind and sun. I spend hours cleaning my cameras and notice that the Loba people (the natives of Upper Mustang) are always sweeping sand even when there is no firmer substrate to sweep it off of. And everywhere there are caves. Thousands and thousands of caves in impossible places. Whoever dug them must have known how to fly. That's the legend, anyway.

All of them were mostly unknown to the outside world until 1992, when the kingdom opened to tourism. Wherever the caves are easily accessible, they've been looted. During China's Cultural Revolution, Tibetan freedom fighters, called Khampas, were trained by the CIA and used Mustang as their last refuge. Artifacts were lost and sold to buy arms after America withdrew its support. Some locals believe that we're here to continue the theft of their cultural treasures. It's happened before.

Some caves are ancient apartment complexes. A few are monastic hermitages and small monasteries with frescoes painted on the walls. And some are burial crypts. The oldest generation of Loba believes nothing should be disturbed, especially the dead. We balance belief with archeology and science and make every promise to be respectful. But mostly people are curious just like us because they've lived beneath the black windows forever. Our assignment is an archeological mission to unearth the mysteries of the grottoes and climbing is the only way to access the secrets because, sadly, everyone has forgotten how to fly.

Matt Segal is a tiny red dot high on an expanse of orange sandstone that looks like vertical mud. The loud buzz of a hammer drill echoes off the canyon walls. He makes slow progress, drilling deep holes into the crumbling rock and hammering in long pieces of rebar as he climbs. Above him are seventeen dark caves that look like big airplane windows. These caves are said to be an ancient library and powerful Tibetan monks levitated to access them, which makes sense because I can't imagine how else they'd get there. Maybe scaffolding? Maybe the gorge has eroded 150 feet in a thousand years?

Matt reaches the ledge outside the library complex and I'm bending over with my back to the wind, trying to change lenses. I don't hear the rock fall but I do hear something hard hit something hollow that sounds a bit like a dropped watermelon. The scream that follows can't be faked. It's frantic and raw and immediate and shocks every sense to attention and now I'm running.

I see a blob of huddled people. I see twitching and spasming legs and now I see the blood. I watch our videographer, Lincoln Else, shake and convulse and there is foam and spit around his lips. He's combative as sandy hands hold his legs and arms. Now his eyes are rolling back and all I can see is white. His skin is clammy and gray and he's inhaling hard against the back of his throat making sounds like a broken harmonica. Now I'm holding the back of his fractured skull and it feels soft like a baby's. The blood is warm and thick and more black than red. It drips around my hands and through my fingers and into the sand, which is everywhere and sticking to everything.

Cedar Wright is passing a roll of medical dressing around and under my hands and saying, "Lincoln, can you hear me?" but Lincoln isn't home at the moment. Pete Athans, the team's leader, is taking his vital signs and scribbling notes and trying to shine a penlight to see his pupils. Liesl Clark is on the satellite phone to Kathmandu, and someone is saying something about a helicopter as radios crackle and locals chatter in Tibetan and Nepali. My hands feel sticky.

Time doesn't pass but a helicopter lands in a loud rotor wash of dust and chaos and everyone covers their eyes. We huddle over Lincoln and try to keep his head protected and say clichéd things like "You're almost outta here!" and "You're gonna be fine!" The engine whines. We turn our backs. A blast of air lifts our shirts and sends a backpack rolling across the stones and I see the wrapper from a roll of gauze fly away. The rotors *thwock* against the thin air and we watch the helicopter disappear until everything is quiet. I look at my camera and know the sand will never come out.

Back at the teahouse, we sit at the table as Pete talks to someone on the satellite phone doing his best to make sense of how Lincoln is doing. Is he stable? I pick at a small tear in a floral tablecloth and float between hypervigilance and distraction. The helicopter has been grounded. Are all these flowers the same? Are these flowers at all? Or are they blind horses? I go to my room and clean my cameras, using a toothpick to scrape the sand from all the hard-to-reach places.

When I wake up, little pieces of yesterday are everywhere. There's Lincoln's harness and there's a pile of trash with finger smudges and dried blood. There's the backpack that flew away, and everyone looks like they've been awake for a week.

Pete answers the sat phone, nods, and says "Yes, okay" and "I understand" and "Thank you." He hangs up and tells us Lincoln has a 21-centimeter skull fracture but he's stable. I remember his soft head and stand to go grab my cameras because there is still work to be done and the magazine can't publish my excuses. I want an excuse to forget. I ask Cedar, "Hey, have you seen my gloves?"

"You're wearing them."

Over eight weeks and two trips to Mustang, we find paintings and piles of ancient text. Pete and Liesl and the archeologists are relentless and patient. There are frescoes and old pieces of hardwood from the lowlands and beads from Afghanistan. There are knives and bracelets and skeletons with deep cut marks in the bones as if they were skinned before being put in the ground and there is as much mystery as dust.

I've made over sixty thousand images and most of them aren't that good. When just twelve pictures are published, I see the space between good and good enough. For me, good enough isn't because I'm a relentless perfectionist. For the magazine, they're good enough to get a second assignment. But first I have other important appointments.

19

Weddings are basically funerals with cake.

—RICK SANCHEZ, *Rick and Morty*

'm awake before Liv, which is rare, and I stare at her while she snores in little whispers. I notice the bones of her neck. She's kind and graceful and everything I'm supposed to want. I love her thick black hair that spreads out over the pillow. She teaches yoga and has long sinewy muscles and can bend in impossible ways. I love the way she fits against my body, and I think I'm lucky to have her.

When I'm not on the road, I mow the lawn, which is always too dry and makes me sneeze. I fix the fence and Dad helps us build a deck because this is what he loves most. I try to count the number of decks he's built in my life. Five, I think. I tear up the carpet in our living room and paint the concrete white and lay down rugs where Liv does yoga in the sun that comes in through the windows and I watch her from the kitchen. In the morning, we go to a coffee shop called the Laughing Goat and sit under a collection of my portraits from Nepal. They're black and white and printed in rich tones of gray that make the wrinkles and squinting eyes appear three-dimensional.

I sprinkle a packet of raw sugar on the foam of a latte and like the sweet crunch of the first sips. These days, it feels like my brain notices too much and too little at the same time. I notice descending rings of coffee on the inside of my cup and the clink of porcelain and plates and a spoon falls and bounces. Sounds are a bit louder now and all the edges of the world seem sharper. I attribute it to a renewed sense of appreciation for everything because I've walked the edge, tipped over it briefly, and found my way back. It is that. It's also something more. There are other, more subtle things shifting in me that I don't immediately see.

My short-term memory feels fragile and I walk into a room and don't know why I'm there. I'm looking for the keys in my hand. I'm looking for the sunglasses on my face and holding the phone as it rings but can't remember whom I'm calling . . . little grains of sand falling out through cracks. But I sweep it under the rugs in the living room and forget about it because I don't remember doing it. I just hope whatever I'm feeling will fade. Maybe the light shining on me will fill in the cracks. And the light is bright.

There are parasols hung in the cottonwood trees in our backyard. Some are colorful and some are white. Some are large and others are small, and the sky is crisp and blue. Café lights are strung in long lines and the lawn is very green because I've known this day is coming and have made sure to water it. A hundred folding chairs are laid out and it smells like fresh-cut grass. Every person looks more beautiful than the last and many are crying as others smile. Mom is wearing a steel-blue dress and shawl and holds my brother's hand. I'm surprised he's here. The last fight was on a frigid night in Minnesota and we haven't spoken in five years. No punches were thrown but love was sworn off with his hand around my throat and spit in my face. Regardless, I'm happy to see him as he smiles in a way that reminds me of summer days chasing invisible enemies through the willows.

Liv walks down a grass aisle as I stand on a small deck built around a cottonwood tree. I'm wearing a gray suit with messy hair and look down at my turquoise shoelaces. Dad is one stair below me in a gray waistcoat and a new haircut that Mom made him get. He's crying the way he always does when things are beautiful and I notice how blue his eyes are. He stands as my best man.

Someone reads a quote about love and someone else reads a poem and I promise all my senses and devotion and future to Liv, who is stunning in an elegant, simple white dress. We both say "I do" and the officiant says, "I now pronounce you married." I wonder if it's weird for parents to watch their children kiss passionately. We smile to everyone as we walk off the platform.

A friend covers a Ben Harper song that goes, "Forever always seems to be around when things begin / But forever never seems to be around when things end."

I hold Liv tight around her waist and sway while everyone watches and I whisper, "I love you." What I mean is "I love everything about you." For this to last, I know that I'm supposed to love her in some deeper, more encompassing way that can withstand the changes and challenges time will inevitably bring. But I don't. And now it's too late to say it.

This is what thirty-year-olds are "supposed" to do. We grow up and commit and make promises we have no idea how to keep, still very certain about lots of things. With Liv, I felt everything until the feelings started to slip away. Now I don't know where all the feelings went, but I'm praying they'll come back. I look at her again and say, "I love you," trying to convince myself and everyone else.

We honeymoon in Thailand and Liv does yoga on a beach deck where we lounge at night and drink cold Singha beers and burn citronella incense to keep the mosquitoes away. We lay with a candle between us on a low table and I notice her dark skin and the long shadows of her muscles. The light flickers while I stare at her face and feel far away. I can't tell if I'm part of anything or just watching it. I don't know how long I've been staring and these little lapses in time seem to be happening more and more while I remember less and less.

History is full of broken promises. I knew that it could never last but I still said, "I do." I imagine many people have felt this as they bend their hearts to fit the shape of an inherited story of love. I know I'm not the first or the last. It doesn't make it okay. There are many reasons why I've forced myself and I'll uncover them all in time, but the why will provide no relief. Liberation will come from something different.

Forgiveness of others asks that we make room for their humanity . . . which is to say nobody is perfect. Sometimes forgiving ourselves is the hardest work of all because it begins with admitting how we blew it to begin with. But once we accept our innate fallibility, we can begin to admit and concede and speak difficult truths. We must empathize with the pain we've caused and feel our own and anger usually comes first. Make no mistake—you can't bypass the "Fuck you!" on the road to forgiveness, whether it's ourselves or anyone else. Don't mark your calendar . . . there is no timeline. For me, it will take exactly twelve years.

Liv whispers, "I love you," and smiles through the candle. I say, "I love you so fucking much," and my heart breaks a little more. I know some stories will never be true, no matter how often I repeat them. Forever won't be around forever. I knew it under the parasols and I know it now. I'm looking for her hand and realize it's already in mine, trying to hold on to something that's already gone.

20

Never regret thy fall, O Icarus of the fearless flight,

For the greatest tragedy of them all, is never

to feel the burning light.

—ATTRIBUTED TO OSCAR WILDE

Sadie calls and tells me my next story for *National Geographic* is approved. Four months later, Conrad Anker and I are two dots in an expanse of ice, trying to climb the west ridge of Everest.

The route was first climbed by an American team in 1963 in a futuristic leap in Himalayan expeditions. The climbing is complex and challenging, breaking off from the standard route at 21,000 feet and snaking its way around the west shoulder of the mountain until it gains a long ridge. From there, it traverses left onto the north face and ascends a tight couloir just below 28,000 feet. It's as remote a route as Everest offers, which is the reason why it's never seen a second ascent. That's why I'm here with the best.

I've known Conrad for many years now. I've memorized his long, lumbering stride and the way he stares and takes time to complete his sentences. He has piercing, narrow eyes that squint like he's always looking into the sun. The right side of his jaw is bigger and squarer than the left side and I wonder if he grinds his teeth when he's making life's harder decisions. He has a narrow smile and balls his fists and closes his eyes tight and says "Yeahhhhhhh!" when he's excited.

Our team arrives at base camp in early April and there is much to do. This is my second assignment and I am carrying a mammoth workload of "deliverables" and I check in with Sadie every day and send "dailies"—images of yaks and the landscape and team. I try hard to make sure she's getting everything she needs while still being a climber and good partner to Conrad. But I'm bothered and tense and scared.

The first hurdle of the climb is the Khumbu Ice Fall. It's a maze of stacked ice that moves as fast as 4 feet a day. The only way to access Everest's upper slopes from Nepal is to climb through it. Tall cliffs of ice break and fall and erase little pieces of the trail daily. But getting crushed doesn't scare me because that death would be quick and painless. I'm terrified of the hanging glaciers on the slopes above the icefall. My body and brain are in revolt because all I can imagine as I sleep and eat and drink and take a shit is the avalanche that is sure to come the moment I stand underneath. The avalanche will not kill anyone but me because it's not a different wall of snow but the same one that I escaped two years ago. I imagine it as vengeful and watch myself get swept away again and again.

When an avalanche breaks free somewhere near base camp, I jump. I'm startled by the roar of an airline overhead. A falling rock explodes and the glacier underneath me pops and I see myself being swallowed whole. I can't sleep on the nights before I have to go up and wish to get sick or for a disaster to strike or for World War III to break out so that I don't have to climb. I hate it with more venom than I've hated anything ever. But there is no one to tell and nowhere to go and nothing to say because I've fought hard to be exactly here. And yet it feels like everything is just a repeating cycle of the same experience and somehow I'm

THE COLOR OF EVERYTHING

trapped in a memory and the past is also now; I'm just wearing a different outfit. I put on my climbing face and step into the darkness, praying to something while I stand in the smoke of the juniper we burn every morning before wandering up.

Only fourteen mountains in the world are higher than 8,000 meters, or 26,246 feet, which is just below the altitude of a commercial airline flight. The average summit-to-death ratio combined across all fourteen peaks is a little over 4 to 1—which means about 22 percent of the people who attempt an 8,000-meter mountain die. Himalayan mountaineering boasts one of the highest mortality rates of any sport.

Adventure storytelling trades on the proximity to death. By virtue of the grim potential, the experience becomes life-affirming and the story goes like this: The hero is disrupted and unsettled and something calls them beyond the horizon. There is a mountain that must be climbed. A sea to sail. There's an adversary to be confronted and death and ruin are the consequences of failure. Inching closer to the edge, the view broadens. The hero sees that in order to understand the world and their place in it, they must traverse the fringes of mortality. Having survived, they find that life is more complete. They understand the enormousness of everything by becoming small. On the journey and in battle, the hero accesses the infinite by confronting their finitude. They understand the mystery of significance by coming to terms with their own insignificance and return from the voyage changed. Across faiths and mythologies, stories of suffering and transcendence are ubiquitous.

This is also a cautionary tale: The hero returns from the edge, but "regular life" feels like a muted continuum of long seconds stacked upon one another and the hero feels called back toward the threshold. But what they seek isn't where they left it. So, the hero climbs a bit higher, goes a bit deeper into the jungle, or voyages deeper into the sea. They risk more, certain that being an inch closer to the edge will broaden their understanding. They endure and survive and their hubris swells.

Over time, the hero begins to mistake the pursuit of the edge for life itself because that's the only place where they feel anything at all anymore. They confuse arrogance with courage, justify their pursuit as a quest for truth, and rejoice as the world fawns. But rather than respecting the divine, they begin to mistake themselves for it, no longer truly believing in their own mortality. They no longer respect the mystery and reject the truth they've already learned. The soldier returns to war one last time and Icarus tempts the sun. The climber goes back to the mountains searching for the highest one.

We celebrate triumph when the hero succeeds and just as quickly criticize when Icarus's wax melts and he falls to the earth after flying too close to the sun. A dark piece of us wishes it upon them. The German word for the dark celebration of misfortune is *Schadenfreude,* a combination of the words for "harm" and "joy." We feel pleasure and even rejoice in the failure of others. If you're being honest, you know exactly what I mean. And yet, if we're open to it, there's value in the hero's fall. A heap of melted wax is a lesson for everyone. I look up at the mountain above me and know that I'm no hero, but I'm definitely flying too close to the sun.

It's just after dawn and the world is blue. My breath is thick steam and my toes are a little cold and there is a thin layer of frost on my jacket. It's achingly beautiful, but I've forgotten to notice. A line of climbers snakes its way through a series of wide black crevasses separating ice cliffs that look like slices of bread falling from an open bag. The cracks are too broad to cross with ladders and the only way around the slices is underneath the hanging glacier I've been dreaming about.

I'm frustrated, scared, and angry because I can't pass the line in front of me. We're too slow and, in my mind, it's only a matter of time until the hanging glacier collapses.

A piece of ice falls above us and explodes into the familiar cloud of an avalanche. Everyone in the lineup frantically looks for a place to hide while I scramble behind a large boulder of ice next to a Sherpa who's mumbling a prayer. The air blast stings my face and neck as white dust washes over us and the only prayer I can think of is "Fuck, fuck, fuck!" I'm uncertain of how big the avalanche is and if we're all about to be shoved into crevasses and buried. Time stretches as I wait to find out. Two years from now, sixteen Sherpas will die where I'm standing.

But the wall of snow never comes, just the cloud. As soon as it settles, the line resumes walking as if nothing happened. I feel alive and I'm confused when I hear myself let out the yelp of someone who's having a good time at a party. I feel renewed and refreshed and the fear is gone, replaced by the feeling of having escaped something.

A week later, Conrad and I are staring up 2,000 feet of blank ice as plumes of snow curl off the west ridge. He coughs and rubs sunscreen on his face. The climbing isn't technical, but the year is dry, and the slope is bare ice that shines and looks gray from a distance. We call it "bulletproof" because it's ancient and hard, compacted by eons of melting and freezing.

The ground is too steep to walk but not steep enough to climb, which makes the movement awkward and cumbersome. There's nowhere to rest and nowhere to stand and everything makes me mad. My big red space suit is too warm and I'm sweating. Conrad mumbles something about blue-collar conditions and I grunt.

We're tired and hot and my eyes sting from sweat and sunscreen. The watch says we're at 21,600 feet. Camp 2 is 1,000 feet below us and we stop and look at the colorful little city of bright tents.

"What do you think?" I ask. Conrad looks up at the massive couloir overhead, which seemed so much smaller from below. This path was my idea and is obviously not working. He looks across the gentle slope that intersects the ridge lower down and answers, "These conditions are slow," which is a nice way of saying "This was a bad call."

We're a few paces apart and I'm squinting and shifting my weight from one foot to the other so my calves don't cramp. Conrad is cleaning his glasses while I put on ChapStick and something hisses overhead. It's thick and orange and a little bigger than my torso and I see the rock in slow motion as it careens between us and whistles down the slope, bouncing and smashing into the ice. I watch it until it disappears and one of us says, "Fuck!" A rock that big going that fast doesn't knock you off. It doesn't break your arm or your leg. It goes right through you. My chest feels heavy and my breathing is short and we start down-climbing without talking.

Back in Camp 2 an hour later, I notice my breaths are still rapid and shallow. I strip off my down suit and someone puts a stethoscope on my chest. They listen for fluid in my lungs and someone says something about a pulmonary embolism and someone else mentions heatstroke. A doctor straps an oxygen mask to my face but I keep breathing and everyone is talking about me like I'm not there. Nothing feels wrong but nothing about being here feels right either and a piece of me wishes I'd never come. The radio crackles and a voice says the safest call is to evacuate. I'm embarrassed and relieved and confused all at once. I'm not sure what's real and what is pretend and whether I want any of this, no matter how hard I've worked to get here.

After a frantic descent through the icefall with Mark Jenkins, the veteran *National Geographic* writer assigned to the story, a helicopter lands. I crawl in and huddle on the seat next to Sadie and take long deep breaths from the wet oxygen mask. The rotors shove us upward and we fly into a white wall of clouds that obscure the mountains, making them seem too close. The helicopter whines and protests and we dive through the clouds in a steep circle and my stomach fills my throat. Fifteen minutes later we land in a village called Lukla and Dr. Luanne Freer puts her arm around me as I climb from the helicopter holding the bottle of oxygen in one hand while pressing the mask to my face with the other. My climbing boots feel clunky as we cross the tarmac in air that feels too thick.

The hospital bed is hard and the walls are green and cold. There are electrical nodes stuck to my chest and an IV in my arm and Luanne hovers over me. "Well, your chest sounds just fine and your heart seems good, so I'm just going to give you a bit of morphine." In one minute I'm warm. In two minutes my breaths are slow. In three minutes I'm asleep. In four minutes it's dark and marvelous and I never want to wake up because I want to escape the truth of this day forever.

I'm in Kathmandu two days later clicking through scrambled TV channels when the phone rings.

"How's the patient?" Luanne asks.

"I feel good. I don't know what happened. I think I can go back."

"Cory, I think you had a panic attack."

The truth is messier.

The brain is marvelous and malleable. It is at once durable and delicate and a universe unto itself. It's the only place *you* exist and it's evolved to protect and survive by whatever means necessary. Sometimes it short-circuits.

Trauma is inescapable but it's also widely misunderstood. Trauma isn't an event but how the mind responds to that event and how that shapes our behavior moving forward. It's also incredibly important to understand that while the memory of trauma is stored in the brain, it's stored in somatic memory as well—it's in your body.

It's also become an abused buzzword, so it's important to understand the difference between the garden-variety trauma of good ol' livin' and post-traumatic stress disorder (PTSD).

It's often (but not always) acute and/or life-threatening events that lead to PTSD and there are volumes written on what it is and why and how it happens. And yet for all the research it's still a bit mysterious. When confronted with an extreme threat and/or stress, a deep piece of the brain called the amygdala is triggered and we fight, freeze, or flee. Most often the prefrontal cortex, the piece of the brain responsible for thinking and planning and regulating stress, shuts down the acute stress response when the threat is over. But after an extreme event, the hippocampus, which is responsible for memory, can convert the event(s) into a long-term memory in an attempt to avoid the same situation in the future. Once the long-term memory is locked in the brain, both the amygdala and hippocampus are resting on hair triggers.

A myriad of triggers that often seem unrelated to the event itself can ignite the hippocampus, which communicates to the amygdala and we go through the stress response all over again. Individuals with PTSD begin to live as if their lives are under imminent threat. The prefrontal cortex is constantly overridden, no longer able to regulate the stress response. Over time we become less capable of dealing with even the simplest of life's challenges because the part of the brain that's responsible for rational thought and future forecasting is basically offline. With memory and thinking malfunctioning, we live in the danger of the past and the present becomes unlivable as the brain is screaming,

"Survive! Survive! Survive!," unaware that it's killing us with stress.

Culture often reserves the label "trauma" for events like combat because of the meanings we attach to those experiences. But the brain doesn't distinguish between an explosion on the battlefield and rape and getting T-boned on your way to work and an avalanche. Culture validates trauma based on its source and we pass judgment on what matters and what doesn't. But PTSD is an *unconscious* response and the brain is indiscriminate. It doesn't care about the story of how it happened. No one's PTSD is more valid than another's. Trauma wears many masks, but to the brain and body it's faceless.

We lose memory. We get angry because nothing makes sense. We dissociate. We withdraw. Life blurs while the brain spins like an unending top. Joy is replaced by a dull hum. We drink and fuck and swallow pills and smoke all sorts of things to dump water on a brain on fire. We punch holes in the wall and throw our phones at the ground and rip laptops in half and I think this all sounds pretty familiar. I did and do and will do all of these things and immediately feel foolish as I drive to the Apple Store.

We don't know why some people shrug off life-threatening events and others are swallowed by them. Also, it's a bit unclear exactly how much trauma is relative to expectation. If the expectation is that you'll go through violent rites of passage and you hold the belief that it's just a normal part of life, is the likelihood of PTSD reduced? In some cases it seems to be. Conversely, if we believe that violence is wrong and safety is the baseline, does that increase the likelihood of a trauma response when we encounter it? Clearly some events like rape and abuse are much stronger indicators. But did tribes who went to battle as an expected part of life, even a valuable one, experience the impacts less? It's an unanswerable question, but one that deserves a bit of thought. Some research shows that the anticipation of negative outcomes is related to stronger trauma response and PTSD. More research is needed.

Complex PTSD (C-PTSD) is caused by repeated traumas and can be its own tangled mess. It's often more persistent and can take far longer to resolve.

Now there is a fist in my face and a hand around my throat. Now I'm running away and in a different home and now without one. Now I'm dangling at the end of a rope with a hole in my leg. Now there is blood dripping from my hands while my friend's eyes roll into the back of his head.

Because my childhood was so stressful, my mind grew to love chaos and used it as a coping mechanism. Survival is what I know and the pursuit of madness was its own fucked-up safety blanket. But now the coping mechanism has become the trigger itself in an unending loop. In *The Body Keeps the Score*, Bessel A. van der Kolk lays it bare: "Being traumatized means continuing to organize your life as if the trauma were still going on—unchanged and immutable—as every new encounter or event is contaminated by the past."

Eventually I'll learn all the words and articulate the experience of trauma to others. But I won't accept it for myself even as I rip laptops in half and patch the drywall and forget whom I'm calling. At the same time, I'll hide behind it and abuse it, and it will become its own mask and justification and rationalization. For a time, trauma will become my identity. It will be true and false at the same time. I will use it to manipulate and escape responsibility even as I help bring it to public consciousness and validate it. When it becomes a buzzword, I'll see that I've been as much a part of the problem as of the solution. The point is not to rob people of their own experience but to be mindful that we don't abuse the diagnosis and dilute it. PTSD is never an excuse. It just helps us understand behavior.

I fly home and wear a bright blue T-shirt while the local news interviews me on the bench outside my house. I tell the world I had a panic attack. I want it to be so easy, connected only to the stress of the job and a rock falling—something succinct. But I know as I say it that there is a deeper truth.

Turning around on Everest was tied to very real PTSD from the avalanche on Gasherbrum II and I was in deep emotional distress, but it wasn't a panic attack. It was a way out. I was having trouble breathing, but I could've stopped it and I knew it. End of story. I didn't have enough courage to say what needed to be said: "This is all too much. I'm terrified." I make no excuses.

The news crew packs their white van and I wave. Mom calls and says, "It's okay."

"No, it's not."

She thinks we're talking about a panic attack.

"We love you."

I hang up annoyed. For now, I'm the survivor mistaking hubris for courage, unable to see that the most courageous thing can be reduced to a single word: help.

21

As long as you keep secrets and suppress information,

you are fundamentally at war with yourself. . . .

The critical issue is allowing yourself to know what you

know. That takes an enormous amount of courage.

—BESSEL A. VAN DER KOLK, *The Body Keeps the Score*

In November 1975, Angola gained its independence from Portugal and quickly devolved into a bloody civil war lasting twenty-seven years. By the time the explosions stopped in 2002 and the tanks were burned out and the jets were crashed or decommissioned and the walls were all pocked up by bullets, over four million people had been displaced, nine thousand child soldiers and eight thousand underage brides were scarred by horrific trauma, and millions of land mines were left as little secrets in the dirt. Eight hundred thousand people were dead.

I learn all this on Google in 2015, sitting safely in an air-conditioned apartment in Boulder, Colorado.

I learn that the war was hardly about Angolan independence at all. Cuba. The Soviet Union. The United States. South Africa. A handful of nations had used African soil as a proxy battleground that absorbed a sea of Angolan blood spilled out of political self-interest. It was a slaughter justified in the name of patriotism and God, as wars usually are. But this chapter is only partly about war. It's about land mines and termites and a river that runs through them.

I board the first of many planes to Luanda, the capital of Angola, with Mark Stone. On the first flight I sip bad wine and read, absorbing as much alcohol as information, and leave my passport on the plane because I drank too much. I don't remember the next flight.

A week later, I stand looking over the Angolan highlands, where elephants and lions should be. It feels haunted, empty, and vast. This landscape should be flush with big game and predators, but the animals were driven south and butchered for meat or tusks or blown up during the war and everything is eerily quiet.

A woman with an infant slung across her back and a basket balanced on her head hops down the dirt road on crutches, missing a leg from a land mine. I feel lucky and sad and pained and indifferent. I take a picture.

The fat trunks and gangly arms of baobab trees give way to hazy yellow grasslands dotted by enormous black granite mounds that appear like puddles through the heat mirages rising from the savannah and I'm listening to Alt-J: "Three guns and one goes off / One's empty, one's not quick enough / One burn, one red, one grin / Search the graves while the camera spins."

We wait an hour to refuel the jeep and I wonder how an oil-rich country can be so thirsty for gas. When I try to make pictures, people hide their faces or threaten me in Portuguese, weary of cameras in the fog of war. Our white faces are magnetic, and my camera is a beacon of wealth. Sometimes the art of photography is knowing when to put the camera away.

In the evening we bounce past the carcass of a rusty tank and our fixer, Paul, slows to avoid the potholes and washboard. I look at Mark and say, "One more?" "Always." This is our language of taking pictures on assignment. If it might make a good image, we always stop. We pull over and the backlit dust of the Land Rover hovers in a red halo around the machine while a motorbike sputters past and a lone figure in the distance walks from somewhere to somewhere else. I take a picture.

When we rendezvous with the rest of the team, a caravan of reinforced HALO Trust 4x4s smash their way through dense old-growth forest, following an invisible road and referencing military and Google maps to avoid the hidden land mines. These 4x4s are reinforced with a thick sheet of steel designed to protect the passengers from the upward blast of someone else's war. This is the most dangerous area of Angola and has been called "The Land at the End of the World." It has many secrets.

At dusk, the convoy breaks into the fresh burn of a brush fire and rolls down a dusty slope to the banks of a lake. The Cuito River doesn't flow from the south bank because it's not a river or a stream or even a brook at this point. It just kind of leaks into a shallow valley of grass stretching south. And yet this lake and trickle are the source of the beating heart of southern Africa.

Nearly 1,000 miles downstream, the Okavango Delta of Botswana is bursting with life. Big cats and rhinos and hippos and ungulates traverse the wetlands of a pristine wilderness nearly untouched by development. Lions eat zebras, and elephants swim, and the long necks of giraffes twist in the sun.

This unassuming lake to our right is the source of 70 percent of the water that feeds the Okavango, and it feels too humble for what it will become 1,000 miles from now. It feels too innocent for what it will tie together.

The premise of our expedition is to gather enough scientific data to convince Angola, Namibia, and Botswana to protect the ecosystem from the dangers of mineral extraction, damming, and mismanagement that threaten life downstream. But the

$400 million tourist industry of Botswana shares none of the revenue with Angola or Namibia, making the protections a hard sell. It's hard to act inclusively when you're being excluded.

Tents spring up in the tall grass as thousands of pounds of food and gear and instruments are laid out and organized. Eighteen-foot fiberglass canoes called *mokoros* slide from the trailers into the water as an energetic South African scientist named Dr. Steve Boyes barks orders.

Steve is a tall sixth-generation South African with a tangle of salt-and-pepper hair and patchy muttonchops and I can't tell if he shaves this way or if his beard just refuses to complete itself. He's the kind of smart that makes you feel like you should've studied harder at everything. He knows more about the Okavango ecosystem than just about anyone. His eyes are gentle and blue and always seem to be looking downstream even when there's no river in sight.

The following morning a layer of steam rises off the lake and it reminds me of the way snow moves across the winter roads of the American West and I feel far from home. My boat slides into the water and I sit near the front as a Bayei man stands behind me like a gondolier, gripping a long pole called an *nkashi* carved from a mogonono tree. He has a gleaming bald head and makes fun of me in a playful high-pitched voice as I struggle to balance. We call him Water because his given name is too hard for us to say.

Twenty minutes later we reach the outlet of the lake, which is clogged by a tangle of thick vegetation, and I reluctantly dive in and pull the seven-hundred-pound boat through a tangle of weeds and hope that there are no snakes. We make less than a mile of progress before pitching our tents. With no shortage of disappointment, we can still hear clear voices in the camp we left behind.

In the morning, Steve slips from camp in the dark and comes

back sweaty. He tells us that the stream, where it exists at all, is too shallow for floating. Usually it's just a marshy grassland that will swallow our shoes. There are groans and laughter and I hear Mom say, "It is what it is." Everyone attaches a harness to their chest and clips themselves to a branched tether attached to a laden canoe and we begin to trudge forward. The boats drag behind us and my legs scream.

For the next ten days, two teams take turns dragging seven canoes less than a mile a day through razor grass and bogs and heat that blisters our shoulders and neck. Every night we can look back and see where we camped the night before, and 1,000 miles stretches into an incomprehensible mindfuck as we eat rice and beans and biltong and sleep in such exhaustion that I'm surprised I wake up at all. My first thought is, "Thank God." But just as quickly, all I can think is, "Oh, God . . ." I take as many pictures as I can but mostly give up on day nine because everything looks the same.

On day ten, a tight, winding stream finally allows the boats to float but requires us to crawl into the neck-deep flow and hack at the muddy banks in dark tunnels of grass to make room for the canoes. The cuts from the razor grass become soft, white mounds of flesh and I exchange a dry sleep for a wet one and stop counting the hours and days and miles because why? I remember Australia and think so much has changed but this all feels very familiar.

On the morning of day fourteen, I press the small rubbery buttons on the satellite phone and turn my back to the sun so I can see the screen because everything here is too bright.

By now, a three-meter-wide stream is meandering through the grasslands and the water is so clear the boats seem to hover above a bed of soft sand destined for the Kalahari Desert. Unlike most rivers, the Cuito will not flow to the ocean. I wonder how long it will take for the sediment beneath me to reach the flood plains, dry up, blow away, and begin a new life as a dune.

The scientists collect samples while I let the phone talk to space and sprinkle dry tobacco into a rolling paper. It beeps as I light the cigarette and I like the quiet crackle when I inhale. There are two messages.

Sadie is checking in. It's not too late in D.C., so I call and tell her I'm making at least one good image per day.

"I like that. One a day."

I tell her that it's mostly a flat expanse of grass and she laughs.

"Sounds thrilling. Keep shooting."

"Okay."

The second message is from Liv and reads simply, "I've hired a lawyer." My face flushes and my cheeks feel hot as adrenaline rises up the back of my neck and I notice that it's hard to swallow. It's always hard to swallow when I'm scared. I've known this day was coming for four years. My head feels heavy on my neck; I let it hang loose and limp, and I sway. I close my eyes and inhale and remember all the things I'd rather forget.

Liv and I are staying on a lower floor of the Fairmont Hotel across from Benaroya Hall in Seattle. It's gray without rain and I like the smell of kelp and salt and the Puget Sound. I feel at home in this city and tonight old friends will gather to see how far I've come. I'll watch them from the stage, making eye contact and smiling at our inside jokes. It's a triumphant homecoming and I want Liv to be here and meet my old city.

I come back to the hotel after doing a sound check and the door clicks open. "Hi, baby!" I say. But the room is empty and too quiet. Someone honks on the street below. My laptop is open on the table displaying a string of glowing text messages to another woman and a green Post-it with Liv's handwriting is stuck to the screen. I don't read it because I don't have to.

I don't remember the first time I cheated. I don't remember why. In the four years we've been married, I've spent more time away than at home. I've been on assignment to the Himalaya, Indonesia, Myanmar, Antarctica, and the Russian Arctic. If I'm not out making pictures, I'm speaking. All of it has blurred.

If I'm not in a tent, I'm in a hotel and hotels are the worst because no one is looking. There's a minibar and a phone and I can mix the two and conjure flesh. I tell the same story and step offstage. People stop asking me questions. The event ends and the bright lights dim and it's suddenly too quiet. This is where my secrets live like little land mines. Maybe if I'm wrapped tight enough in the arms of a lover, I won't keep floating away, dissociated and disconnected.

Sex is a solution and my therapist says something about a "coping mechanism." As much as I hate this piece of me, I have a hard time controlling it even when I know it's going to cause pain. I like being able to charm a room or a person. I like breaking the monotony of telling the same stories and I love being adored by a stranger when I can't stand the company of myself. I crave stimulation. And when life runs out of adrenaline, I've learned to make it. I give the wheel to the dark sailor and watch him head straight into a storm.

Infidelity is another expression of the chaos I chase. It fills space. It starts with a drink and ends with a shower and now the room is even quieter but I'm quite drunk and sleepy, so I close my eyes and dream of getting caught so I won't have to hold on to the secrets any longer. Ironic as it seems, it's an expression of believing that love isn't for me at all.

In Seattle, I stand on the stage in front of twenty-five hundred people and pretend everything is okay. I hope my friends aren't there. If they are, I hope they can't see my red eyes as I tell stories of virtue and perseverance and discovering truth by confronting my limitations and myself. The audience applauds and the room clears. The lights go down and I close my eyes and hold them shut until I can hear the river again.

The sun is very hot now and I feel it on the top of my head. I look at the satellite phone and finish my cigarette as the sounds of the water and birds and voices return. The river doesn't care. The birds don't know. There is literally nothing I can do but float downstream.

At points the river is choked by thick trees and we take turns diving in with machetes while making morbid jokes about crocodiles. This place has a sense of being abandoned and infinite, as if the war eviscerated everything but a grassy shell where life used to be. Hot, silent hours pass, interrupted only by the team counting birds and calling out species as they spring from the banks.

We meet no one, but we know we aren't alone. At night, we see large grass fires set by locals to flush game and make travel easier. The fires are beautiful from a distance and we watch them for hours, knowing all action comes with consequences. Steve tells me the roots of the grass and trees hold the delicate Kalahari sand in place, and once they're destroyed, rainfall pushes the loose soil into the flow of a river system that hasn't evolved to carry it. I take a picture and Steve looks downstream.

He explains that other pieces of the ecosystem have been protected by the aftermath of war. With millions of land mines in the ground, expansion in rural areas halted, keeping great corridors of earth nearly untouched by development and deforestation. The land mines create a humanitarian crisis that leaves people limbless and blind and I think of the woman I photographed on the road. But as soon as an area is de-mined, the forests are cleared for farmland and the timber is burned to make charcoal as a meager source of income. The soil loses more structure and compounds the problem of flood and flow and water.

When we finally do meet people, they speak broken Portuguese through tribal dialects. Most of the communities have no real contact with Angolan society and it's hard to reconcile that Luanda, the capital, is the most expensive city in the world now. Oil and diamond money pours in by the billions while entire communities are forgotten and I think it's funny how shiny things can make it very hard to see.

When we run out of meat and break an axe, we follow a trail through the bush and trust the path is safe. After two hot, itchy hours, we stumble into a village that hasn't been visited since the soldiers came through forty-two years ago. Steve tells me these people are Luchazi, and I take a picture while villagers crowd the hut door to watch the tall white man with blue eyes negotiate and listen and take notes. We buy two skinny chickens and an axe.

After a month, we reach the town of Cuito Cuanavale and collapse into the dusty breeze-block bunkers behind the HALO Trust headquarters. We dry out and smoke and take the opportunity to drink as much as we can. It's mostly warm beer and I try to hold off until dinner, but whiskey at noon is my favorite.

I pitch my tent in the shade of a storage shed and try to sort out my divorce via satellite phone and half listen to the lawyers while editing pictures. The attorneys are fighting and one mentions "the value of your client's photographs . . ." and another says something about the fairness of "leveraging art as poker chips in a game of matrimonial chess." I sweat and think of their air-conditioned offices while I use a twig to scrape dirt from under my toenails and try to calculate the actual "cost" of infidelity. It's not about the dollars. It's the emotional cost and I feel selfish as I contemplate how much the pictures I'm looking at are "worth" in the context of a marriage. It seems disgusting to even think it and it's all compounded when I open an email from Liv and it says something about narcissistic personality disorder.

———

We all have narcissistic traits and a heightened expression of them is not necessarily psychopathology. But as I research it, I'm scared because many of my actions do reflect a heightened degree of narcissism. I'm horrified that I'm adding a new set of complications to an already complicated brain.

Narcissism, like trauma and PTSD and ADHD, has become a pop culture buzzword. Research indicates that the rate of clinical narcissistic personality disorder (NPD) remains consistent, with the disorder affecting about 1 to 6 percent of the population. Narcissism is often used to help people explain the source of profound pain and abuse in relationships that were undoubtedly toxic. It sucks to feel fooled by someone when they fuck up or turn out to be different than we'd hoped. Whether we were intentionally manipulated and cheated or not, it feels that way.

Pathological NPD presents as an encompassing self-perception that is all-powerful and knowing, gorgeous, influential, and entirely infallible. Like most psychological dysfunction, NPD is almost certainly tied back to some sort of developmental trauma and emerges as a maladaptive survival mechanism. It's also essential to understand that the grandiosity of narcissism is actually a mask for shame and self-hatred. A clinically narcissistic person develops these traits over time, and they don't come and go. A narcissist might choose maladaptive behavior later on, but they didn't choose to be a narcissist. As hard as it can be, it's best approached with compassionate accountability. Sadly, someone suffering with NPD will often reject it all the same. Likewise, it's incredibly hard to diagnose because a clinical narcissist is likely to avoid therapy or psychological evaluation that might challenge them. It's also extremely important to remember that as tempting as the story of narcissism might be, not all toxic relationships mean that we were with a narcissist. Sometimes we're just mismatched and end up being awful to each other.

The outsized confidence of NPD can be and often is confused with the grandiosity of bipolar disorder. The difference is that bipolar grandiosity abates once the cycle of mania or hypomania is regulated. The bipolar person can and does feel real regret, shame, and guilt. They can see and do understand how their actions have impacted friends and loved ones and they feel genuine remorse. For a bipolar person, the masks of infallibility will fall away and they'll reconnect and concede. Sadly, those admissions can viciously amplify cycles of depression. That said, neither bipolar nor NPD is an excuse for being a flaming asshole.

Both NPD and bipolar people have higher rates of infidelity. Both are characteristically impulsive. So for Liv, the story of narcissism makes perfect sense to explain my actions. It's confusing business and I understand why. But when I eventually address it with my therapist, frightened that I now have another mountain to climb, she calmly says, "Cory, you are many things. But you're not a narcissist."

"Just a moody, selfish dumpster fire?"

"I heard that was just added to the *DSM*."

The distinction for her, and for me, is that my grandiosity and impulsivity come in waves and I'm sorry for it all, even if it takes time to get honest. The big difference is that narcissists intentionally set land mines for other people to benefit themselves. It's calculated behavior and they often know they do it. Bipolar people tend to step on the land mines that fall from their pockets while they're manically running through a field.

I do feel regret and carry guilt and have deep remorse for all the pain I've caused. I feel shame, however useless it is. I don't think I'm any more special or beautiful than anyone else even if I do like to look in the mirror from time to time. By this point in the book, it should be clear that I don't think I'm infallible or perfect.

As for empathy, the bipolar mind seems to be at a disadvantage. It's ironic that individuals so profoundly influenced by heightened emotional states are the same ones who have a harder time recognizing and empathizing with the emotions of others. Research in this area is scant and there isn't a clear answer to why. For me, it doesn't come naturally. It's not that I can't be empathetic . . . but it will take time and the tears of many more before I begin to learn it. When I finally do, I will be frightened by the fires I set.

But for now, looking at my dirty feet and listening to the lawyers fight, I'm fearful of myself, confused by my own actions, and angry, though I don't know at what. My only release is the story unfolding around me and the river below, carrying me further downstream in an unstoppable current of life.

The tourist outpost of Maun is a half-paved swirl of faded dust choked by Land Rovers, helicopters, and tiny airplanes that buzz and hum like mosquitoes. Sun-bleached curtains hang from always-open windows, open-air cafés play reggae, and beer is measured in liters. By the time Mark and I arrive, we've been in Africa for almost three months. I'm tired and wet and shriveled and dusty and speaking fewer and fewer words to anyone. Conversation requires energy and energy requires rest and we haven't stopped in months.

While we plan an overland tour of the delta to photograph the ecosystem at risk, we stay in a hotel and draw the blinds and sleep like we're dead. I edit and eat and drink many liters of beer. I do push-ups. I talk with lawyers and think about divorce and write ill-advised, reactive emails and scan the thousands of pictures I've made, looking for holes in the story and solving how to fill them. A portrait of Steve surrounded by a cloud of determined sweat bees says more about the expedition than words ever can. Somehow, he still seems to be looking downstream. There are pictures of erosion and landscape. Poverty and opulence and war and violence. Destruction and regeneration.

Six days later, I sit in a small helicopter with no doors, pointing the camera across the delta. Banks of long green grass wave
on the edges of winding channels that shape round yellow islands. The water seems too clear to be real. Thousands of deep
ruts are worn into the landscape by millions of paws and hooves
in an enormous knot of life. Herds of elephants, buffalos, and
zebras splash and throw dust. Giraffes move in single file and
cast long, skeletal shadows and I wonder how long it took to
make a path and how long it will take to disappear. Lions and
crocodiles sunbathe. Leopards sleep and chew on limp limbs of
prey in the shade of acacia trees while hippos surface, snort and
grunt, and then disappear as if annoyed at the world.

From above, tiny pale termite nests pepper the islands like
scattered ash. From ground level, the termitaria rise as high as
17 feet and look like mud candles.

Steve tells me that termites are the "architects of the Okavango" because their colonies are responsible for the 150,000 islands that make up the ecosystem. As a nest grows, sediment
brought by the floods collects around it, making it bigger with
every season. Eventually it becomes a small island. And because
the mound provides a high perch for birds and mammals alike,
they sit on top and drop seeds in their excrement. The seeds find
purchase and roots stretch out under the soil and catch more
sand from the floods and the islands keep growing.

But before they build, termites destroy. They feed on wood and
grass and break down other life until it collapses from the inside
out. I wonder how many living things have been devoured to
make the islands grow.

In relationships, secrets are termites that feast on intimacy,
self-value, and trust until the raw material of love loses its structure and disintegrates. Whatever Liv and I shared was eroded by
dishonesty until it collapsed on itself. That I'd known it would
never last was the biggest lie and perhaps even a subconscious

motivation to destroy it. It wasn't calculated, but all the secrets I carried made it impossible for me to love and be loved. I made many mistakes and now I'm looking across the delta at the landscape destruction built.

If we get honest, the wreckage of secrets can guide us toward safe harbor if we're brave enough to stare into ourselves and understand what we hide and why. The secrets we keep are the pieces of ourselves we deem unlovable. But when we embrace them, they lose their potency and no longer hold power over us, releasing us downstream, and I think I know why Steve is always looking that way. Downstream is the future, and if we choose honesty, the future is always hopeful. We're never outside the reach of rebuilding and forgiving the mistakes we've made upstream. It's frightening work but worth every mile we travel. With enough time and courage, the mistakes of our past become the unshakable bedrock of a better future.

Eventually Liv and I only communicate through lawyers and after the ink dries on all the divorce papers I'll keep a nice set of knives and the rights to all my pictures. We'll never speak. I'll apologize when I finally understand, but that is a ways downstream. Sometimes a pain is too deep and a betrayal too much. Sometimes it's just easier to forget than forgive. Often we can't understand the depth of a wound we've inflicted until it's been carved into us.

The day we leave the delta, my eyes are red, dry, and stinging. Mark and I pile into the truck and I bow my head and close my eyes, covering my face as we drive to the dirt airstrip. I've made all the pictures I can and spin them backward and upstream in my head all the way to the picture of the tank 1,000 miles ago. It was dusk then and everything was red. It's dawn now and everything is blue.

The road is bumpy and I taste sand. A tall, proud termite mound with the trunk of a dead tree suspended in the mud stands like a monument of decay and rebirth. I look at Mark and say, "One more?"

"Always."

We stop and wait for the sun. Today photographs are what I have. I don't know what direction I'm looking, but I hope it's downstream.

22

Being crazy isn't enough.

—DR. SEUSS

The TV is on, but I'm staring at a pair of fake eyelashes on the windowsill. I don't remember where they came from but I see that they've been there long enough to collect dust. Divorce is confusing. In death there is finality. In divorce the living become ghosts and it's easy to be haunted. Africa was brutal and illuminating. As difficult as the whole process was, I came home tired but hopeful and ready to move on, but moving on will take time.

I live in a small apartment with gray floors and east-facing windows and everything is new aside from the knives. The cupboards close quietly and the floor is silent when I pace in the kitchen. It's light and lonely all at the same time as I try to navigate from isolation to solitude. I don't know what comes next. But I do need to pee, so I guess I'll do that. It's the little things.

I think the mirror is being an asshole because the reflection I see is familiar but vague, as if I'm buried under some puffier version of myself. There are toothpaste splatters and water stains and loose hairs in the sink. I look pale. I need to clean. I need to shave. I need to wash my hair. I need to go outside. I need a win. I'm sorry, mirror, you're not an asshole. You're just being honest.

There are days that I don't leave the apartment and watch TED Talks between champion bouts of *Family Guy* reruns while looking at my phone and willing it to ring. Life isn't bad, it just feels empty, like I've lost something and I don't know what it is or where to look. It isn't just the void of my marriage but something deeper and formless.

Depression is sneaky and sometimes we only really see its depths once we climb out. It's hard to realize how deep you are when you're transfixed by the crumbs on your belly. I also feel a strange sense of guilt for being depressed at all and at the same time it feels impossible to escape. People of all walks of life have experienced deep despair; some people just have to get up and work in spite of it in order to survive. I know it could be much worse and I feel more guilt that my legs just won't move. Telling a depressed person they need to get out and be active is like telling an insomniac they just need to count some sheep and go to sleep. I look at the eyelashes again.

On Tuesday the phone finally rings and Adrian Ballinger asks, "What are your plans this spring?"

I don't even have plans for the rest of the day. "I don't know," I say. "Watch *Family Guy*?"

I've known Adrian for a decade. He's handsome with dark features, light eyes, and freckled skin that's seen too much sun. His ears are big and his cheeks seem stretched between his angular jaw and cheekbones. He's relentlessly optimistic and laughs loudly and often and loves coffee. We like to call him "Stick," which is short for "Stick Bug" because he's tall and skinny, and I can vaguely see him on the other end of the phone when he says, "Do you think it's time?" I know exactly what he is talking about but look at my watch anyway.

Four years ago, after far too much alcohol and too many hours awake, we'd made a plan. I'm listening to his British-Boston accent bending *r*'s into *w*'s and staring at myself in the mirror with the phone to my ear. He's talking about climbing Everest without oxygen and I'm happy he can't see the body I'm living in.

The toothpaste splatters block one eye and Adrian waits for an answer. Before fat Cory can say anything, athlete Cory hidden underneath speaks up and says, "Yes." I pause. "But I'm, like, chubby and smoking a lot of cigarettes."

"You have until April."

The next morning I call my friend and mentor Steve House and ask if he'll step in as my coach. He's one of the best and most respected Alpinists in the world, and if anybody can give me a shot at this in three months, it's him. He agrees and I hang up the phone and then go to the gym and stay there for three months. I bike or walk up hills slowly, keeping my heart rate below 150 beats per minute while breathing through my nose. Steve says it will increase my aerobic capacity and mentions something about "fat adaptation." I think I'm fat enough, but he explains that the term refers to teaching your body to use its fat stores by training fasted on long endurance days. At altitude it's hard to eat, so it's important that my body knows where to look for energy when I've run out of candy bars and burned through my love handles.

I've called myself a professional athlete for a decade but I finally understand what it means. There's no glitz aside from crawling into my bed knowing that I trained as hard as I could. The only glamour is sleep. There is no time to smoke or drink or fuck. But because there is a light at the end of the tunnel, I'm more hopeful because I'm driven by purpose. A certain amount of loneliness is necessary in the service of an objective. It's different from the vacuum of depression. I think if I'm going to be isolated either way, I might as well use it as a space to grow toward something.

Some days I'm embarrassed at how slow I have to walk to keep my heart rate low. When I do burpees, my torso jiggles, and I check the mirror every morning for bigger muscles and a smaller belly. Steve tells me to be patient, to train slow to go long, and reminds me, "It never gets easier, you just get faster."

I wake up at 5 A.M. and pull on long wool socks and insulated running tights and stack on all my warm layers. I fill collapsible jugs with gallons of hot water for added weight in my backpack and scrape thick ice off my windshield without gloves and think of Dad. I listen to AC/DC and Rage Against the Machine while driving through the darkness to the trailhead. When it's snowing, my headlights make the flakes fly past in streaks of white and it looks like I'm in *Star Trek*. On these days, the trail is empty and I see no one for hours. They are the same trails and the same day over and over and over.

When it's too cold to train outside, I spend five or six hours on the treadmill with a backpack, reading *King Leopold's Ghost* or *The Looting Machine*. Sometimes I watch *Game of Thrones* on my phone and fantasize about marrying Daenerys Targaryen. Who hasn't? Anything to pass the time. Anything to keep my mind occupied. When I'm frustrated, Steve calmly reminds me that "it's better to be consistent than talented" and I say, "I'd like to be both." He laughs and replies, "Wouldn't we all? Control what you can. Fuck the rest of it."

My legs get faster. My heart rate goes down. I climb 9,000 feet on Monday and 11,000 on Tuesday, Thursday, and Friday.

After three months my muscles aren't any bigger, just tighter, and I'm disappointed because I look nothing like the men and women I see on the cover of the magazines in the grocery store when I'm buying arugula. I sit on the floor and listen to my brittle tendons crunch as I roll them out and wonder why growth and improvement always hurt so much. The burpees start to feel less like torture and more like release and the crumbs on my slightly smaller belly are quinoa instead of chips. I'd kill a bunny for some chips.

By the time I get on a plane to Nepal in early April, my brain feels different. Everything seems brighter and the clouds of depression have parted around the summit in my head. I wonder if this is how a phoenix feels as I look at the shrinking flames around my feet and hope the lack of oxygen at the top of the world will starve the fire completely.

Two weeks later my neck aches from trying to sleep on a minibus bench that's too short for my body. I study the cracked faux leather of my seat as the engine whines and downshifts up a thousand switchbacks to a high pass on the Tibetan Plateau. Faint scars of an ancient trade route weave their way between the smooth blacktop bends and I open a tattered window curtain and stare at the new road cut. When we round the next corner, the hillside falls away into a horizon of soft, burnt orange foothills, all over 16,000 feet.

Slashes of red stone cut across the hillsides and intersect with the collapsing walls of monasteries that appear to melt more than erode. The shadows are deep purple and the sky is more black than blue. Heaps of tattered prayer flags litter every ridge in dots of red, blue, yellow, green, and white and I wonder who put them there and when.

The pass crests at just over 17,000 feet and I finish my third liter of water at 10:30 A.M. I can feel my pulse behind my eyes because I'm not acclimated and I gasp as I step from the van. The light is flat and muted by a layer of high clouds over the serrated horizon of five of the world's highest peaks. On the left are Makalu and Lhotse. To the right are Cho Oyu and Shishapangma. The four peaks frame the pyramid of Everest rising high above the other summits. Like so many of the mountains I've climbed, it seems too big and it's still 100 miles away. But by now I understand that all mountains are climbed as a series of pieces and either I'll stand on top or I won't.

Two hours later we turn off the main road and follow the flood plain of a turquoise river. The landscape is barren and gray, interrupted by shaggy livestock and yak drivers with long black hair tied with red yarn and patinaed yak bones. They walk slowly with their heads tucked against the wind, clasping their hands behind their backs, whistling and hollering over the sounds of bells and snorts.

The asphalt disappears into sand and I think of all the dirt roads I've driven to a dead end where one journey ends and another begins. Eventually you have to walk. And after you walk, the reward is the climb.

The rolling hills have become shattered walls of yellow stone that rise thousands of feet in columns on either side of the river, which is now just a frozen white line. I feel my pulse behind my eyes again and drink more water because my mouth is drying up the same way it always does when I'm intimidated. At some point on every expedition, I'm unnerved by the remoteness of it all. I've learned the best way to navigate the unfamiliarity is by bending the definition of home, and now, I will do it again. The minibus pulls into a broad, dusty basin dotted by tents and whines to a halt.

After ten days of acclimation, Adrian and I traverse the broken terrain of the Rongbuk Glacier and listen to ice crack and break as boulders crash down from the fresh glacial scar and the ground under my feet feels new. It's broken and unsettled, toppling over itself and uncertain where it fits.

We break left up a sandy embankment where the trail is too steep to accommodate two-way traffic and settle into the slow rhythm of the yak driver in front of us. I smell his sweat and my sweat. I smell dust and yak shit and rocks grinding against rocks and think this place is somehow perfect.

Two hours later we perch on the broad spine of a broken black slate and drink tea while we stare up at the mountain. I see exposed ice and small tendrils of snow swirling off a dark ridge. But the swirls aren't small because the mountain is still 5 miles away and the ridge is 10,000 feet above us. We finish our drinks and Adrian drives us toward advance base camp at 21,000 feet. He walks in long strides and tucks his thumbs in his shoulder straps as I struggle to keep up, questioning if I'm strong enough to do what we've come here to do.

On either side of the trail, countless 200-foot ice towers rise as blue spikes that break and fall and talk to us when we're breathing too hard to speak. When we do talk, it's of relationships and sex and the mountains and our plan. But eventually there's no more talking. We are together but in our own worlds, just like all relationships. When there's no conversation, it's just the labored breathing of high places that reminds me that our bodies don't belong here.

From advance base camp, I trace the line of ascent through a series of crevasses and ice cliffs to the North Col. From there the route angles up and left, following a broad ridge that frames the immense north face. The top is barely visible, hidden behind the mile-long summit ridge, which is the most dangerous part of the climb because it traps climbers above 8,000 meters for so long.

After two days in advance base camp, we start the pulse of acclimating, climbing high, sleeping low. Climbing higher, sleeping low. Sleeping higher. Climbing higher. It's the rhythmic demystification of the Himalaya and the same method I've used on every high mountain. I remind myself that every climb feels impossible until you stand on top. So I memorize the steps and colors of the ropes and crevasses and always try to run under the big hanging ice cliff that guards the saddle of the North Col.

Ten days later, we sit in a hot tent at 23,031 feet and sweat. The interior can get to 75°F during the day and plummet to

−20°F overnight. We drink Soylent, a supplement mix that tastes vaguely like pancake batter, while making Snapchat videos that fulfill our sponsorship commitments and tell the story of the climb in real time.

The idea to use Snapchat as a real-time storytelling tool came from Adrian's girlfriend, legendary rock climber turned Himalayan star Emily Harrington. Now #EverestNoFilter is trending on the platform and hundreds of thousands of people are following the climb. Thousands of messages of encouragement, music recommendations, trolling, and the occasional picture of breasts flood our inbox. The connectivity of social media feels satiating and it also seems to blur and confuse motivation. But social media is ubiquitous now and at times it seems more important than the climbing itself. The premise of telling the story in real time is to offer an unfiltered and authentic look into what an expedition like this takes, but I quietly question how anything on social media can be authentic.

#HairByEverest begins to trend because my unwashed, sun-bleached hair makes me look homeless and Adrian's looks like he's just been electrocuted. People start posting pictures of their babies with wild hair and tagging it #HairByEverest and I like the playfulness of it all.

At 25,000 feet we spend a night in a tent dug into an exposed knoll that falls away thousands of feet on both sides. Adrian watches *American Horror Story* on his phone while I read *The Old Man and the Sea* and listen to the wind whipping the walls. I like little books on expeditions because they weigh less, and Hemingway's short prose is easy to understand when your brain is starving. Eventually we fall into an uneasy sleep.

Just after midnight I wake up and see the wind has drifted hundreds of pounds of snow against the uphill side of the tent. The poles are bowing and threaten to break under the strain. The collapsing wall is hanging inches above Adrian's body, encasing him. If the tent poles do break, they'll rip holes in the fragile nylon and the tempest will be let in. If the wind fills the tent, it will balloon and get blown from the perch, and us with it. If it doesn't blow away, it will shred the fabric, filling the tent with snow and sending the gloves and boots and clothes cascading into darkness, and any safety we have will evaporate. If we don't fix this now, we'll either blow into the void and die or be relentlessly exposed. And die.

When I shake Adrian awake, he looks stunned and annoyed before he realizes what's happening and springs to action. Two minutes later we're outside, furiously digging the drift away, knowing that if the storm persists it will fill back in within the hour and I know that I won't sleep for the rest of the night. I can't. But descending in darkness seems more dangerous than the meek shelter of the tent, so I sit awake and melt water until first light.

When dawn breaks, we crawl from the tent into an angry windstorm that instantly freezes exposed skin. The tip of my nose stings and then goes numb as we hurriedly throw everything we need into packs half filled with snow. I dig out the ropes and start down, trying not to trip over my crampons in a dehydrated, sleep-deprived stumble.

Two hours and forty-six minutes later, we collapse in a heap at the bottom of the route and stare back up toward the tent. But the mountain is nowhere to be seen, swallowed by a strange neon gray.

It's May 24, 2016. I'm thirty-six years old. My alarm goes off at 12:30 A.M. but I'm already awake because "sleeping" at 27,224 feet is like "meditating" at a Metallica concert. Adrian's headlamp comes on first and I shield my face for another minute of staring at the tent ceiling. It occurs to me that I spend a lot of time staring at different ceilings.

Eventually I sit up and start the stove, exhaling clouds that collide with the steam rising from the water. I wonder about matter changing form and how heat can make liquid levitate. Invisible currents make the vapors rise and swirl in the light of the headlamps. I look again at the ceiling and see all my breath from the sleepless night frozen in a sparkly frost. Gas becomes solid. I wonder if the altitude is getting to me and vacantly drag a finger in a line, watching the crystals fall onto my sleeping bag and melt.

I've been awake for eighteen and a half hours, minus the thirty minutes when I managed to hang somewhere between sleep and wake, trying to forget about the sharp stone jabbing my left ass cheek. It will be five and a half more hours before the sun rises. I unzip the door just enough to see the thick stars of high places. My eyes trace along the uneven edges of the last 1,811 feet of Everest's northeast ridge rising above me as a heavy black triangle.

I tuck back in and watch the steam in the tent and remember the past five months and the thirty-six years before that and everything that brought me to this place at this time as Adrian and Pasang and I prepare to leave for the summit. Pasang has joined the summit push for the sake of safety in numbers. Everything is done in silence. I no longer think about which boot or glove goes on first because I know it doesn't matter. The only thing that can get me from here to there is my breath.

We leave the tent together and follow our familiar circles of light. The route climbs shallow snow to a steep series of wide granite cracks that lead toward the ridge. We check in with each other every half hour. Can you feel your fingers? Toes? Are you drinking? Eating? How does your head feel? Lungs? Are you slurring? Are you vomiting? What's your name? Where are we?

Gradually the gap between Adrian and Pasang and me widens and I stop communicating by voice and start calling to them over the radio. After three and a half hours, the space between us has widened far enough that I feel alone and all my concern of not being fit enough has been swallowed up in the darkness. I'm not behind them, but ahead.

Adrian's voice comes over the radio in slurs and tells me that he's too cold and moving too slow to continue. He and Pasang are turning around.

"Are you sure?"

"Yes," he says quietly.

"Do you want me to come with you?"

"No. Keep going."

The communications are short and labored. But this was always the plan. If one of us couldn't and the other was still strong, we'd separate. The team's doctor, Monica Piris, who's monitoring our climb from advance base camp, takes over the conversation. She's spent many nights just like this, sleeping on the uneven floor of a dining tent curled up next to a tangle of cords and radios and solar batteries to keep it all going as her team plods through a dangerous and foolish darkness. It's her job to keep us safe, to keep us moving, to keep us alive regardless of whether we're climbing up or down.

I half hear her voice as I fumble with a rope. "Adrian, I need you to get back to the tents at high camp as quickly and safely as possible. When you're there, please put on oxygen to get the blood flow back in your hands and feet and brain." An indistinguishable mumble, half wind and half words, fills the air and I realize that Adrian is riding too close to the edge.

"Are you sure you don't want me to come down?" Mumble. Monica answers instead. "Cory, how do you feel?"

"Good. My left pinky is tingling."

"Keep fucking going! Adrian and Pasang will be safe. Go now. Go fast. I'll talk to you in half an hour."

The radio goes silent and I turn off my headlamp and sit. I

listen to the breeze brushing across me and feel the wet collar of my down suit against my face. I am alone. I have no oxygen and no backup and no safety net other than my body and an honest accounting of myself. There are five other climbers somewhere on the route, but I can't see or hear them. My life is apprehended in the confluence of breath and wind.

An hour later I approach the legs of a lifeless body hanging upside down in a tangle of rope. Tufts of loose feathers push through the torn suit, fluttering. I think of Marko and Daria and Peru and the little girl who pushed me and my camera further into this life. I think of all the friends and people I've known who are no longer and lose count because my brain is too slow. I think of all the bodies I've seen on this climb and all the others in various states of decomposition and wonder again at matter changing form.

Sometimes they have faces. Sometimes they have mustaches and beards and eyelashes. Sometimes they're hooded and hidden, as if they're sleeping. Other times they have fingernails and their exposed flesh is yellow and black. Their skin is freeze-dried against bones that stick through, mummified after they took off their mittens in their final delirious moments. Their body and brain became confused and lied, telling them that they were warm and safe to shelter them from an opposite truth. Hormones and chemicals saturated their minds, creating a definitive hallucination to comfort them as they took their last breaths. This is the agreement you make with high mountains. Here the sliver of space that separates life and death is immediate, implicit, and yet totally incomprehensible.

My fingertips scream from cold as I unclip myself from the rope, reaching over the body and connecting myself to the line on the other side. I take a single step and walk further into life than the body behind ever made it.

When the sun finally rises, the summit pyramid is washed in

fluorescent pastels and my pinky doesn't tingle anymore. I take out my phone and try to film, annoyed at the intrusion. But the battery dies from the cold, and I'm relieved that the final steps will be just for me.

I don't know how much time passes between this and the moment I sit down on the summit. An hour? Two? When I take the final step, there is nothing and no one and literally everything on earth is below me. I reach as high as I can and touch space. There is no place left to go. In some fundamental way, I've exhausted the search outside myself for anything that might make me whole. But I can't see this now. For seven minutes I sit in silence and my awkward mind is literally the highest point on the planet.

After forty hours without sleep I walk into advance base camp. The air feels thick and humid here. My heartbeat is slow and my mind is too tired to race, unable to comprehend the place I've been and how something so powerful can be so brief. I'm exhausted but restless and forget to go to bed. The world already knows what happened because, up until the final steps, they'd watched me. For his part, Adrian is as outwardly excited as everyone else but I can see how much he wanted it and how much it hurt to fail so publicly. I can see how much humility is required to let me shine. The depth of his character is revealed behind his skinny, chiseled face. He is more resilient than I ever could be.

A week later we're in New York City and 2.3 million people are watching Adrian and me, with slightly gaunt eyes and sunburned faces, sit across from Gayle King on *CBS This Morning*. I wonder if the cameras can see the dry flakes of skin peeling from the tip of my nose. Later in the day, we sit across from Charlie Rose at his iconic wooden table and tell the story of the climb until he refocuses the conversation on what I'd disclosed about my mental health.

Just before the summit push, my anxiety peaked. I was overwhelmed by the climb, attention, and exhaustion. And, because there was no one else to talk to, I told a million people on Snapchat because that's what the world does now. I'd matter-of-factly disclosed that I was bipolar and anxious and depressed and that everything was getting to me. I talked about being scared of the climb. Scared of failing. Scared of being scared and what that meant. Sending the videos into the world, I'd wondered if I was oversharing in the pursuit of attention. But even if I'd wanted to recant, it was too late. By morning my public persona had begun its transition into a spokesperson for mental health and the story behind the now infamous self-portrait from Gasherbrum II was slowly seeping out. Private became public. Superhuman became human. And, through the conceit of "no filter," something mysterious became less so, inviting everyone into a much more real experience.

So when Charlie asks, I open up and speak candidly about the avalanche, PTSD, and bipolar because it seems natural. I can feel that it's somehow important to break down the wall around me.

More interviews and TV follow. More press. More questions. More answers. When we finally unload a heap of tattered duffels on the curb at Newark Liberty International four days later, the expedition has generated over two billion media impressions. Two billion eyeballs.

I say goodbye to Adrian and Emily and walk to the gate, equally relieved and uncertain to be flying "home." The word has shapeshifted again and I feel far away from the mountain, where things were less noisy, less frantic, more basic, and more meaningful. Where coffee tastes better because it is the end and not the means. When the nice lady in a silk scarf with wings on her blue lapel leans over my seat and says, "Welcome home, Mr. Richards," I wonder what she means because home is somewhere in a tent where the only planes are the ones that fly overhead and up there the captain is saying, "If you look out the window to your left, you can see Mt. Everest."

After the divorce, the success of #EverestNoFilter is intoxicating. I float through days and weeks and am filled up when strangers thank me for speaking so candidly about my brain. While climbing Everest without oxygen is special (less than 2 percent of summits), it's not new. It's been done. For me, the accomplishment and celebration seem to be centered around something else. Suddenly my weaknesses are being celebrated as my strengths and I wonder if Achilles might have lived forever if he'd taken more care of his heel. And still I'm filling the inescapable space inside of me with the mountain itself because from it I can speak truths that I've held on to for too long.

I also know once the shine wears off, an emotional deflation will ensue and the comedown will be equal to the high. The next four years of my life will be devoted to trying to regain the same summit. I'll stand there again, but it will never be the same.

23

The dark does not destroy the light; it defines it. It's our

fear of the dark that casts our joy into the shadows.

—Brené Brown, *The Gifts of Imperfection*

'm in Colorado and Jeremiah Fraites pours me wine, looking a lot like Woody Harrelson. I would describe him more, but that's the most efficient way. He's wearing a white T-shirt and black pants with suspenders. Aside from his lace-up black boots, I'll never see him in anything else. His wife, Francesca, checks a pot of spaghetti, which is also the name of their dog. Francesca is a small, native Italian spitfire with long jet-black hair, pale skin, and fine red lips. Fra never minces words and is unafraid of her opinions, the way all Italians are, and tells me the story of how she ignored Jer when they met. She makes clear that he was *her* groupie and not the other way around. Jer chuckles and shrugs because it's true.

They do the dance that all couples do in kitchens, weaving in and out of each other amid steam and dirty dishes and wet counters. I envy an obvious, real love that allows for living side by side without needing to fill the space that always exists between two people. Jer scrapes vegetables into bubbling marinara and wipes away tiny red dots of splatter as quickly as they land because he cooks as meticulously as he makes music.

The wine in my hand feels awkward as I tell him that I drink too much, which is obvious in my cheeks and eyes. I swipe a piece of thick bread across my plate to soak up the last of the sauce when Jer asks, "You wanna hear something?" Of course I do.

I pour more wine and follow him and Fra into the basement and turn left into a cave. There's a guitar in the corner next to a stack of notes and scribbled lyrics on a bookshelf and I feel like I'm in *Almost Famous*. It's dark and a mess of keyboards, microphones, and wires clutters the desk. A dim lamp is casting a yellow triangle of light across the face of an old upright piano that stares at us from across the room and the keys look like a broad, toothy grin. Jer says, "You have to promise me you won't tell anyone," and I cross my heart and hope to die as he hands me headphones and taps the keyboard. His face glows bluish white as he scrolls down through files and folders. Fra holds a Polaroid camera and takes pictures with big flashes. Jer doesn't look at me but says something. I lift the headphones off one ear. "What?"

"The new album. It's called *Cleopatra*." He taps the space bar. A high-pitched drone whines into a slow, thundering kick drum and the world disappears. When Wes Schultz's raspy voice cuts in, I start to cry. I don't stop for thirty-four minutes.

Maybe it's the alcohol and exhaustion of living so hard. Life feels so fast these days. Maybe it's hearing a friend's art or feeling that what I'm making isn't enough. Sitting next to real talent and fame can be as shattering as it is intoxicating.

We listen to the album and every song seems to have a piece of me in it. Wes sings, "But you held your course to some distant war / In the corners of your mind."

I rest my face against my hand and try not to ugly-cry. Jer is beating at the drums and tapping the piano and Wes keeps singing: "Fate / Dealt you a tricky hand / Now you're just left alone in your mind."

The music stops and I'm overcome. My face is still in my hand and Fra takes a picture, freezing the moment and a shared piece of us. I've always looked for moments just like this in my own photography but now I feel exposed, realizing how much I ask of the people I photograph. The Polaroid will hang for years on various fridges and walls as we braid in and out of each other's lives. Jer smiles and laughs. "So it was all right?"

"It's nuts," I reply, which seems like a clumsy thing to say. We sit quietly for a few minutes before he gets up and makes his way toward the stairs. He stops and stands above the piano and fingers the keys to "Ophelia" and I ask, "Do you think I'm an alcoholic?" It comes out of the blue, but this has been on my mind lately and I want someone to answer for me. His T-shirt stretches over his hunched back, and I can see the mound of his spine casting a shadow. "I don't know, man. Are you?" He knows there is only one person who can answer.

I'll come back to this night when I feel safe and unjudged and secure enough to be insecure. That's what deep love and friendship offers. We always have the answers to all our questions. Even in the noisiest mind, we always know. Finding answers isn't hard. It's speaking truth that takes effort. I crawl into the car and think I've probably had too much wine and drive home in silence. I want to hold on to the melodies as long as I can, aware of how much music has always held me.

Laurel Solé has sandy blond hair and soft, blue eyes that always look a bit tired. There are furrows at the end of her eyebrows because she is always thinking and watching and interpreting. Most of all, she listens. Her movements are quiet and deliberately gentle, and I wonder if she's always moved this way or if it's something you learn when you become a therapist. She enters the office, closes the door gently, sits, sighs, says nothing, and smiles.

I lie on her couch against striped pillows. There's a table and lamp with soft orange light and a box of tissues. By now I've killed a forest in rooms just like this. Maybe my next sponsor should be Kleenex.

I watch a squirrel on a branch outside the window and say nothing. The leaves are green and full and I'm clutching two paddles, one in either hand. Laurel instructs me to close my eyes and I notice how hard it is to keep them shut. My vision has always anchored me to the world, pulling me outside of my own inner landscape. I'm startled by her voice when she says, "Now, I want you to remember . . ." and the little paddles start to vibrate, alternating from right to left.

In 1987, eye movement desensitization and reprocessing (EMDR) was developed to treat PTSD. It's guided by what the therapists call adaptive information processing, which aims to unravel and reprocess the emotions, thoughts, beliefs, and physical manifestations of trauma—to release the memory from the hippocampus so it stops fooling the amygdala into reacting. The focus in EMDR is on the memory of the traumatic experience, changing the way it's stored through bilateral stimulation. The best working theory is that by stimulating both lobes of the brain, traumatic memory can be integrated, shifting us out of the sympathetic nervous system into the parasympathetic and reengaging the prefrontal cortex. In order to fire up both lobes, they use eye tracking from right to left, or tapping, or the two miniature vibrators in my hands.

With my eyes closed, she asks me to think about my brother. Because there is not one experience but many, the memories appear as shards. We're screaming and there is the hand on my neck and a white flash from a fist. There is speed and tears and a door that closes behind him as the words "I don't love you. I'll never love you" hang in the air. My stomach begins to convulse, and

loud sobs become silent as violent contractions constrict my dia-
phragm so that no air can escape. Whatever sounds I do make
are animal and I hardly recognize them as my own. My back
arches and my toes bend and curl as the arches of my feet begin
to cramp. I wonder if I'll shit myself on her couch because my
whole body is flexing, trying to release something held so deep
that it seems to have no source. Just a bottomless well. This is an
exorcism.

The emotions are confusing. As much as there is pain and
anger, there is also guilt and shame. A piece of me knows that
I've told my story with outsized blame. There's a depth of honesty that I don't want to admit. It's the part of me that knows that
as real as my trauma is, I'm partly responsible for it. Try as I
might, I can't fault my family for everything that happened and
I know that there's an ownership that I've not dared name. Once
I learned that conflict generated attention, I fed into it, creating
chaos as a way to feel love.

I don't know how long I cry because I'm in the past. There are
shapes and colors and faces and forms and it seems to last longer
than it should. But eventually the crying abates and I have hic-
cups. My back relaxes and my heart slows and a creamy, warm
sensation spreads over my body. This session is over. I open my
eyes and feel embarrassed for crying so hard. The outside squirrel
is gone but everything else is the same.

I come back twice a week for months. Some sessions we only
talk. But Laurel seems less interested in where it all comes from
versus how it feels in my body. She asks me to describe every
sensation. Do they have colors? Textures? Do they have faces and
names? What does it physically feel like? Too much coffee? Electricity? Where is it? My chest? My ankles? My throat? Do I want
to run? I tell her about the women. I tell her about the alcohol. I
tell her that I'm concerned about both and without looking at
her I ask, "Am I an addict?"

"Are you?"

Over the next months, she asks me to remember many things. "I want you to go back to being in treatment as a teenager. . . ." I see LifeLine and blue chairs and faces of kids that appear hollow and drawn. I see a barren, dead landscape in winter and burned grass in summer. There's the hot lunchroom and burritos with cottage cheese inside and fist-shaped holes in the walls. I see my parents crying as I slip into the darkness through locked windows. I see coming back and losing my shoes and belt and shoelaces. She says, "Go back to the avalanche. . . ." I see a white wall of snow and fear and anger. I hear the sound and feel the blast of ice and everything is chaotic and churning. I feel myself cry but am unaware if they are new tears or the ones I cried when I turned the camera on myself. She asks me, "How far can you go back, Cory?" But there is no bottom. It's just a road that evaporates into smaller and smaller bits of memory. Gradually the pieces are too small and I stop crying in the treatments and mistake the calm for resolution.

It's believed by many that if you can heal the "original" trauma, the behaviors will stop. So why am I still drinking and carousing my way through life? I know why I do it. I think I know what happened in my past and the mechanisms of pathology. These stories are concrete now and I can describe them without thinking because they have become rehearsed. And still the story feels incomplete and inauthentic. I'm too certain of many things, and the symptoms aren't abating. There are simply places that self-knowledge can't touch.

My head is a ball of yarn. First it was depression and anxiety, explained by attachment theory and genetics and turmoil. Then it was bipolar, which looks a lot like ADHD and often masquerades as narcissism, all tied to C-PTSD. Then it was a string of additional experiences like big falls and avalanches and near misses, all further complicating my brain's wiring and thinking and patterns. It's so knotted that I'm unsure if it can be undone. I'm pulling at some threads while ignoring others. I'm weaving new narratives of the same brokenness I'm trying to escape. For all the effort, none of it seems to be arresting the behaviors and patterns that seem to be pulling me apart.

24

Reality is just a crutch for people

who can't cope with drugs.

—ROBIN WILLIAMS

I buy a home in Bozeman, Montana, with red hardwood floors and adobe walls. Hops and ivy tangle around the crossbeams of a veranda and a tree grows from a hole in the deck. A long, reclaimed railroad beam supports the second floor on pillars of wood and it's perfect. A reading nook underneath a big window is accessed by an antique library ladder and I picture myself lying in the sun reading with an imaginary woman with long slender lines. Another window opens up to a large backyard where deer wander at night. I'm certain that here I'll be happy and home.

I move all my things from Boulder and imagine a new life with new people who only know me as a question mark. Boulder is done with me and I'm done with it. For a moment I feel calm and whole.

My life feels loud. I have four agents, a publicist, and an athlete manager, all growing my "brand." I have one agent named Sara, and she puts me in front of the camera and onstage as a speaker and helps my other agent, Rachel, who puts me behind the camera as a photographer and in ad campaigns that use my face to sell adventure and cars and rain jackets. She works with two other agents named Stacy and Gina, who manage my archive with *National Geographic.* My publicist, Meghan, makes sure that I'm getting interviewed and on magazine covers, which makes my athlete manager, Caley, very happy. Because it's all too much for me to keep track of, I have a two-person management team named Dre and Malou, who keep my schedule and book flights and forge my signature on contracts when I'm not around. I have two passports so I can get visas with one while I'm using the other, and it's one big machine. I adore all the people who manage me and I'm grateful but sometimes entitled because it's quite easy to forget how privileged I am. This has become normal. In four years I will have no agents.

In the broadest context, to call what I've experienced "fame" seems silly, even though it feels big. Just like with Gasherbrum II, after the media blitz of #EverestNoFilter, the frenzy has slowed and the living room is quiet. The gray couch stretches underneath me as I bend my head up and sip whiskey. It's 10:30 A.M. Despite beginning to unravel my past, I'm anchored to it, guided by the forces I understand but can't counteract. I'm hovering in the space between understanding and action.

It's Saturday and there are seven of us when someone hands me some MDMA that he's had in a bag with some LSD. The night's cold and star-filled as we light the campfire. The euphoria of the drug starts to kick while I make pictures, fingering the texture of my camera and running my hands through my hair, wondering how anything can feel so marvelous. Twenty-four empty cans of beer are stacked in a neat pile and we're passing a bottle of wine around the fire, shaking from the cold and chemicals while every star pulses with great streaks of light. One by one friends disappear into the darkness and the laughter fades until it's just two of us and a glow of embers.

I take another pill and sit in a tiny home built on the bed of an old pickup until everything is just us as brothers and big ideas. I stare through him, tonguing the roof of my mouth, studying the undulations of my skin and the smooth veneer of my teeth because I love the way the world feels. Slowly, white bands of dried ash appear in streaks painted vertically down his face. His dark skin becomes redder and his cheekbones widen and rise and there are feathers in his hair. I stare as his lips ask, "Are you all right?" but he isn't talking. The moisture in the bag with the acid and the pills has mixed the two and I am hallucinating. I'm certain it's a sign of something sacred and true. It's religious. I'm connected to everything and everything is perfect and soft and the hum that never goes away is suddenly silent. I feel every muscle in my body relax as it's never done before and I want to stay here forever.

Eventually his face changes back as the high starts to wear off. I want more. More of the feeling of connectedness, more love, more of everything. It's a desperate need for the night to never end and the feeling to never stop and I want to clutch it, but there is nothing to hold on to.

On the following Monday morning, I'm deeply depressed and there is nothing sacred or divine. MDMA, also known as Ecstasy or Molly, enhances the release of serotonin, norepinephrine, and dopamine and blocks its reuptake. Specifically, serotonin is vital to the regulation of sleep and pain, mood and appetite, and basically everything that makes us feel good. Normally, the brain releases the neurotransmitters in a slow, regulated seep, keeping us level. MDMA causes a torrent. In certain doses and in the right setting, there's strong evidence that it actually helps heal trauma and rewire neural pathways. But in unregulated doses, especially when combined with alcohol and LSD, you have a flash flood of serotonin that's followed by a drought. Dump all that into a brain that's already deficient in serotonin and dopamine, and the comedown is like jumping from an airplane without a parachute. It can take days before the brain bounces back. On Tuesday I want to die.

By now I've done many drugs. Cocaine. PCP. LSD. Painkillers and other pills. But never has the free fall been so complete. The impact has never been this hard and now I'm standing in front of the mirror screaming at myself, saying, "Why are you like this!" The thoughts and emotions speed up and the black-and-white flashes in my brain come back. The hum is a roar and I'm on my knees, tearing at the hair that felt so soft. My mouth is dry and I'm scared of hearing voices. I've been told my whole life I'll go crazy and fall hopelessly into addiction. Is this that?

On Wednesday I'm fragile. Maybe it was just this experience. Maybe this is normal. Maybe I don't have a problem. Maybe this was just once. It's a losing battle against my higher self.

It's amazing how long we can know a truth before we accept it, living in fear of what it means if we finally give in. What will I have to change? What will I have to give up? How many friends will I lose? How bad is this going to hurt? No matter how miserable a situation is, it will never compare to the misery of rejecting what we know is true for us. When our actions aren't in alignment with our values and beliefs, we're living in what's called cognitive dissonance and it's a vessel for more of the same bad medicine. It makes me thirsty.

It's a worn-out cliché that the first step is admitting you have a problem, and it's true for most that in order to break an addiction you must see the problem clearly. You have to see the mountain that needs to be climbed. Tragically, for many it's seemingly unclimbable. Admitting you have a problem means nothing but compounding shame and guilt unless you're willing to climb. It will be steep and hard and exhausting and you'll likely fall and end up in a heap. Maybe you'll get hit by an avalanche.

You're likely to give up at least once, taken over by some invisible force, and you'll watch your hand reach out for whatever it is you're addicted to. You won't want to, but the muscles are working on their own. It will be bewildering when you take the first sip or hit when everything tells you not to. But once it's in you, there's no turning back. You've had one. Have a thousand more. Fuck it.

I'd argue the first step is when you understand all of that and choose to climb the mountain anyway. But because the standard narrative of addiction is "once an addict always an addict," you're stuck in a new story of brokenness and powerlessness that arguably reinforces a negative self-perception. Now you're sick again, and even if you view it as an illness, like cancer, it's incredibly hard to separate from identity. If that's the story you're telling, you're not on a mountain at all but on an unending hill.

I lie on my back and stare. Tears pool in my ears and I finally answer my own question. I name this pain addiction even though a piece of me doesn't believe it. An even bigger piece of me isn't at all ready to quit. But for now it's a useful story. It will help and harm me and I will tell it for many years.

On Thursday I wake up, find my passport, pack my bags, and drive to the airport. I love flying because no one is looking and I can order as much alcohol as I please. No one pays any mind because on planes and in airports, drinking is excused and understood at any hour. I drink until I'm tired and wake up in Singapore hungover. It seems playfully cruel that my next assignment for the magazine is photographing "the world's happiest places."

25

A smile is a curve that sets everything straight.

—Attributed to Phyllis Diller

In 2016, Singapore is the happiest place in Asia despite the threat of public caning for graffiti and spitting. I stand in a neat yellow square on the sidewalk as I smoke and notice the absence of cigarette butts and gum on the pavement. Tall high-rises tower overhead, bisected by perfect streets, manicured hedges, and neat sidewalks. I sweat and wonder what makes this place so happy.

Back in the hotel lobby, Dan Buettner sits across from me and sips a beer. He's tall with a handsome round face, blue eyes, salt-and-pepper hair, and the kind of wrinkles that make him look like he's spent most of his life smiling. He does not laugh but guffaws in a way that fills any room.

"I was so excited that I'd be working with you! Tell me about Africa." He redirects: "Tell me about Everest!"

Often people who have gone on big adventures share an un-spoken bond similar to soldiers who never fought together but know the smell and taste and labor of foreign soil and the dirt that never really comes off. It's not a respect for the person neces-sarily, but the sweat they left behind. Dan left a river of sweat when he biked 11,855 miles along the spine of Africa. After that he dedicated his life to finding and unraveling the secrets of lon-gevity, identifying the enclaves of society where people forget to die. He calls them Blue Zones, and, unsurprisingly, longevity and happiness often overlap.

Like all writers, he's thoughtful with his words and slowly the conversation turns to the job at hand. Dan explains that *happiness* is the wrong word but *life satisfaction* doesn't translate on news-stands. Happiness is a better story.

The first thing he explains is that it's slippery and elusive and I feel vindicated in my confusion. Happiness is both internal and external. It's choices as much as hormones as much as environ-ment. It's how much you walk (lots), how much time you spend with friends and community (four to six hours a day), and what you put in your mouth (mostly plants). It's security and family and ownership and belonging. It's purpose, play, place, and peo-ple and I'm becoming more and more confused by what happi-ness actually *looks* like. Pain, suffering, despair, and war are far easier to photograph because they're immediate and obvious. Dying polar bears and impossible climbs are shortcuts to the limbic brain and humans are uniquely designed to love drama. I've spent years making struggle into something beautiful, but now I'm being asked to make something ethereal tangible.

Dan also explains that the pursuit of happiness often has an inverse effect. Too often we mistake someone else's definition of happiness for our own. We chase someone else's bliss because we think it will make us happy. Or, worse, we buy into a socially curated picture that doesn't belong to anyone at all. Instead, it's an airbrushed six-pack, an overflowing bank account, twenty-seven million Instagram followers who just adore how cute you and your partner look on a yacht in Aruba or living in a Sprinter van in the desert or wearing fairy wings and goggles at Burning Man.

Relentlessly pursuing happiness can subconsciously reinforce discontent because the story we're telling ourselves is that we *aren't* happy. In short, the pursuit is defined by what's known as a "scarcity mindset." A study in 2011 concluded that "valuing happiness was associated with lower hedonic balance, lower psychological well-being, less satisfaction with life, and higher levels of depression symptoms."

The chase reminds us that what we have isn't enough, especially when we equate happiness with the external . . . and in particular with money. Capitalism itself hamstrings happiness by replacing the present with the dollar. Sure, you'll be happy for a moment when you get the boat, the partner, and all the money and sex in the world. And with enough resources, you can chase this external happiness indefinitely. But the best research says that after about $75,000 a year, more money doesn't equate to more genuine smiles because trying to find happiness in "having" or in someone else's version of it is like chasing the horizon: you might end up where you were looking, but you'll never recognize it because your eyes are still fixed outward. Likewise, as much as wealth is often seen as a conduit to greater happiness, it's actually generosity that makes us happier in the long term. Giving, not having, is the gateway to joy.

Dan tells me that end points are hollow and process is full, and I think this sounds very familiar. It's ancient wisdom repackaged. Some new research tells us that imagining a feeling of happiness, especially during meditation, starts to shape our lives toward it despite no external factors changing at all. The pretty people in Venice, California, call this "manifestation," but ironically, it usually isn't about genuine contentment with what is but rather is focused on what we want. The Buddhists, Taoists, and Stoics have been quietly asserting for a couple of thousand years that lasting happiness is about presence as much as it is about where you end up.

The language of happiness has evolved over time. In Middle English it was *hap*, which is the fortune that life offers up, both good and bad. Hap is unforeseen circumstances that unfold from the mystery. It's our lot. Moments of joy are found when we step into the arena with that fate. Knowing that these moments will come and go alongside blistering pain, loss, and heartache, and accepting that and choosing again and again to get knocked down and covered in dust—that is where what we call happiness lives. That *hap* has become *happiness* is part of the problem we are trying to solve.

I watch Dan's face contort. No one can make anyone happy and he knows this. Instead, his job is to uncover the components of contentment and give people the outline of a fulfilling life. My job is to make the blueprint into pictures. How anyone builds the house and what they put in it is up to them.

"So basically, it's a crapshoot," I quip. Dan guffaws because he thinks I'm joking.

I'm invited into a home and photograph a beautiful young bride having her makeup done while family and friends scurry about and a toddler on the floor gums a plastic ring, drooling with joy. Long-term relationships are correlated with greater life satisfaction because commitment fosters responsibility, accountability, and structure. Being dependable and making choices that serve others and getting outside of ourselves give us purpose. A hand with a makeup brush reaches into my frame and the bride closes her eyes. A golden hijab is wrapped around her hair. I take a picture.

I'm in a sea of pilgrims and devout practitioners in a Hindu temple. It smells like sweat and spices and smoke. A bell rings, cutting through the murmur of voices and car horns outside. A shirtless devotee wrapped in a crimson robe laughs. There is a correlation between faith and happiness and I wonder if he is happy. I take a picture.

Six seniors in the park flow through languid tai chi postures and breathe through their noses as meditation and movement are combined. I take a picture.

Women cook together and a man makes traditional dragon masks and people at a comedy club spit out drinks as a trans-gender stand-up comedian shatters Singaporean norms and tells jokes about getting laid. Somewhere, in all of this, happiness lives. I show the comedian an image and ask, "Are you happy?" The reply: "When they laugh!"

On the way back to my hotel, I duck into a neon world that smells like sour alcohol and bad perfume. Tourists call this place "The Four Floors of Whores" and a mean-looking European with silver teeth and sleeves of tattoos ducks past me as I step into a bar through a beaded threshold. The room is washed in blacklight and the world appears as neon clothes walking them-selves. In some fucked-up way I wonder if photographing dark-ness will make happiness easier to see. There are four other foreigners spread throughout the room and no one really looks like they're having a good time. A girl with glitter on her skin sits down. She tries to talk but I don't have anything to say and she finally walks away when she understands I don't want to pay for her affection. I can see that chasing contentment is shining a confronting light into my shadows. I can see that in some way, chasing the picture of happiness is eroding my own.

Back in my hotel room, the girl I met on Tinder kisses me in the meaningless way of a one-night stand and leaves. I hear the door close behind her. It's three-thirty-something in the morning and I already have a hangover. There are smears of makeup on the pillows and sheets and a dirty towel on the floor next to some mini bottles. The light is too yellow and I sit on the end of the bed naked and wonder what happiness looks like. I'm thirty-six years old. I have a gorgeous home and a little bit of gold in the bank. I travel and make pictures for work. I've climbed the highest mountains and my face has been on T-shirts and beer bottles. I'm the first and only American to do this and that. I speak to big audiences and everyone tells me I have the best job in the world. I'm respected. I have ten fingers and ten toes and a nose. I can walk. I have privilege and opportunity and resources. I have security and love and support and friends. I have everything and I'm on assignment for the biggest publication in the world telling a story of happiness. And still, somehow, I'm the unhappiest I've ever been.

The minibar is empty now. I call room service and order two beers, open my laptop, type "rehab" in the search bar, and pass out.

26

You know you're an alcoholic when you

misplace things . . . like a decade.

—Paul Williams

The plane bounces and I wake up under a low ceiling of clouds. Mounds of dense jungle and fields crisscrossed by major roads spread out below me as a flight attendant motions to my seat and tells me we'll be landing in Bangkok shortly. I'm sweating and can feel the imprint of the pillow on my cheek. Blue shadows give way to gray darkness and I don't know if it's getting dark or light and it feels like I haven't known for a long time. I used to love the time warp of travel. I loved the haze of landing in a new place that was either in the future or the past from where I took off. I don't love this feeling anymore.

The terminal is too bright and my eyes sting. It seems like an extravagance to go to Thailand for rehab, but it's actually the opposite. The Western healthcare system makes inpatient addiction care so expensive that the cost is prohibitive for the majority of people who need it most. Thailand is the only place I can really afford.

I board the flight to Chiang Mai and swallow a benzo to settle the anxiety that always comes with a hangover. I swallow an antidepressant to battle the low clouds. I swallow a mood stabilizer to keep me somewhere in the middle and fall asleep again.

An hour later, I wander out of another airport. A woman with sandy blond hair and blue eyes holds a sign with my name on it and we make eye contact. I nod shyly, a little embarrassed that she already knows more about me than I want anyone to know. She greets me warmly and says, "You made it! Congratulations!" with too much excitement. She's used to addicts stumbling off flights, often still high from the last bit of heroin or coke in their system and needing a little extra energy.

"Are you high? A bit drunk? Hungover?" she asks, too matter-of-factly.

"Maybe a bit of the latter. Why? How bad do I look?"

She laughs. "Last week I picked up a guy who had to be wheeled off the plane because he'd tried to drink off his withdrawals. Everyone likes to get a last bit of fuckery in. That's normal."

The roads are a braided mess of scooters, tuk-tuks, and horns as we drive our way from the airport to the facility. I'm anxious and everything feels too hot as I sweat in the front seat and try to make small talk. The main gate is 20 feet tall and made of thick bamboo, supported by a rusty orange steel frame, and the perimeter fence reminds me of a zoo. A broad wooden door with the same magnetic locks of my childhood buzzes and I walk into a new home that separates whatever is inside from the outside world. A nurse in navy scrubs takes my blood and I choose a Hello Kitty Band-Aid and surrender my pill bottles. I surrender my phone and anything else that might distract me.

"Anything else, mate?" a doctor in khakis asks. I shake my head. "Good on ya. Welcome to the Cabin. We'll have ya right in no time. How long er ya stayin' with us?"

"Twenty-eight days."

"All the beds on-site are full, so you'll be staying off-site at the Villa. Go get some rest and we'll see ya tomorrow morning." He pauses briefly, then adds, "You're gonna do great!" He seems uncertain and I wonder if he says that to everyone.

I get up at six, take a shower, and apply enough bug spray to kill an elephant before wandering to an open-sided lobby. I stand nervously and drink bitter instant coffee while a gaggle of other men trickle in. One is Indian and three are Australian. Two are from the States. One is British. One from Singapore. One has been here for ninety-two days. One was here last year but needed to come back. Another says it's his first time here but fourth time in treatment. One is a judge addicted to meth. Another is a lawyer who loves speedballs, gambling, and getting high-end prostitutes when he's on a bender. One is a carpenter, and another is the heir to an international shipping conglomerate. Actor. Musician. Father. Son. Brother. All ages. All walks of life. All of us clinging to the idea that somehow we can be happier.

As anyone who's been in rehab or sat in AA meetings will tell you, addiction doesn't give a fuck who you are. It doesn't care what you do or where you've been or what you've done. I know this because the billionaire's son with no teeth reminds me. We're an unlikely collection of people who would otherwise never meet, all in various states of disrepair and dishevelment. Shaving is the least of your worries when you're trying to kick a heroin habit. No matter how much you pay for luxurious surroundings, recovery is hard, and if you think it's easy, you're probably not really serious about it.

A rugby player with cauliflower ears and a missing tooth points at me while looking at everyone else and says, "Who the fuck is this?" A bearded man with more ink than arms puts his hands on my shoulders and says, "Welcome to the Villa! You're one of us now and we are fucking Villains!" Now I know what the high fences hold inside. I feel like I've passed some rite of initiation while the other inmates laugh and grumble. One man with pale skin and stringy, long hair seems deaf, staring out from a darkness that's obscured all light. A covered truck with open sides pulls through a locked gate and honks. Rugby guy screams, throws his tea on the pathway, and says, "Let's go get unfucked!" and we all pile in.

The program has three fingers—mindfulness, twelve steps, and various modalities of psychoanalysis—and I settle back into the familiar language of institutionalized life. "Issues" and "trauma" and "triggers" and "family of origin" and "coping mechanisms" and "acting out." "Moral inventory." "Powerlessness" and "manipulation." Familiar tropes of recovery flood back in: "You can't bullshit a bullshitter" and "It works if you work it" and "One day at a time." We hold hands and the chorus goes, "God, grant me the serenity . . ."

On day two I sit on the lawn while drips of sweat tickle my sides and back. An American therapist with a gleaming bald head and big, round muscles walks me through the basic premise of cognitive behavioral therapy (CBT) as I sit cross-legged and pet the grass. "Are you listening?" I nod. But after thirty-four years I'm very tired of therapy.

He tells me the method works by confronting the core beliefs that trigger our reactions. Here, they teach the process as the ABCs . . . Action. Belief. Consequence. It looks like this: *Someone cuts in line to the bathroom (action) and I say "Fuck you!" in my head and decide the day is a wash and I should probably have a drink (consequence) because everyone sucks.*

I jump from action to consequence without blinking and I'm living in a fantasy that's become an emotional reality. But something happens in between the person cutting in line and "I'll take a double, Johnny." The brain interprets the action and I tell myself a story based on the subjective life experiences that have shaped my beliefs. If I can catch myself there, there's potential to change the outcome. The method is threefold: Acknowledge the emotion prompted by the action. Question the belief that's driving it. Change the consequence. CBT doesn't focus on how the beliefs are formed but instead works to challenge and change them in the moment.

If I can slow my brain down, I see why someone jumping the line annoys me. This is where mindfulness comes in. Sure, it might be rude if it's intentional. But that assumes it is . . . which I don't really know. Maybe this guy ate a bad oyster and has explosive diarrhea. Regardless, why am I so pissed off at something so trivial? Extreme as it might seem, the message I received is that this guy doesn't value me. He thinks he's better than me. The belief, simply put, is that I don't matter. But it's not his belief. It's mine.

To observers, neurodivergent minds appear extreme and irrational, with a penchant for catastrophe and drama. It's what we know. People with coping mechanisms like drugs and alcohol love a good calamity because it reinforces our stories and worldview. Those stories give us an excuse to indulge. But even in the healthiest brains, most of our reactions and responses can be boiled down to a few core beliefs about ourselves.

But I'm also beginning to wonder if this is a disease of the heart as much as the mind. Can anyone really think their way out of this?

Psychology has long focused on the mind as the nucleus of behavior and it's understandable why. It's been seen as our body's command center. But what this view has missed for so long is the heart's role in the troubled and healthy brain alike. As it turns out, the heart isn't just a metaphor used to describe the vestiges of human emotion.

In 1995, Stephen Porges put forth polyvagal theory, which suggested that the physical heart plays an essential role in social behaviors. The base theory focused on the vagus nerve as a source of "information" that guides social bonding behaviors by influencing heart rate variability (HRV). HRV refers to variations in the interval between beats, and a higher HRV has proved to have positive effects on well-being and social adaptability. Furthermore, the ability to regulate HRV positively influences the ability to judge the emotions of others more accurately as well as increasing sensitivity to social feedback. A study from 2022 takes it even further: "Mathematical modeling of physiological dynamics revealed that emotion processing is prompted by an initial modulation from ascending vagal inputs to the brain, followed by sustained bidirectional brain-heart interactions."

Simply put, in some ways, emotional processing begins in the heart and is sustained by a conversation with the brain. How the heart informs and might even be foundational in consciousness is the next frontier. Neurobiology seems to be proving what our ancestors always knew: The heart itself is the heart of the matter.

The therapist's voice brings me back to the world: "Are you still listening? Do you understand?" I'm silent, still petting the grass, but nod. Conceptually, I get it. Unhealthy beliefs drive thoughtless reactions. Healthy beliefs foster thoughtful response. All actions and emotions are precipitated by a story and that story can be changed. That's work no one else can do and it doesn't get done by simply talking it out or quitting the drugs. The actions of others are not relative to my value. No one gets to decide that story but me. Nine times out of ten, people just don't see the line. And if they do, trust me . . . this shit isn't about you. It might just be bad seafood.

After fifteen days I feel cleaner and clearer. I open an email from Sadie and she tells me they've given the remainder of the happiness story to another photographer. I'm both hurt and relieved that they've assigned someone else to finish the article. That I failed on the story is one idea. That I did the best I could with what I had at the time is another. I wonder if both can be true simultaneously.

I'm sketching during an hour of art therapy when the therapist hands me *Touched with Fire: Manic-Depressive Illness and the Artistic Temperament* by psychologist Kay Redfield-Jamison. Several pages are dog-eared, and the words are biting:

> The great imaginative artists have always sailed "in the wind's eye," and brought back with them words or sounds or images to "counterbalance human woes." That they themselves were subject to more than their fair share of these woes deserves our appreciation, understanding, and very careful thought.

I think of my life in the boat and sailing in the wind's eye. No small piece of me has loved being tortured. But it's another story keeping me stuck. The trope of the "mad genius" is as dangerous as it is romantic.

It's hard to trace the link between creativity and mental illness, but it's clear that there's a connection between bipolar and creative thought and expression. To give you an idea of how common the link is, here's a list of bipolar contemporary artists, celebrities, and thinkers that I found on a lazy internet search: Mariah Carey, Carrie Fisher, Bebe Rexha, Mel Gibson, Demi Lovato, Russell Brand, Brian Wilson, Kurt Cobain, Jimi Hendrix, Ted Turner, Catherine Zeta-Jones, Vivien Leigh, Frank Sinatra, Sinead O'Connor, Jean-Claude Van Damme, Jane Pauley, and Patty Duke. We can only speculate about other names from history, like Vincent van Gogh, Ernest Hemingway, Lord Byron, and Winston Churchill. But the story of the mad genius is as old as time. It also might be a myth.

Bipolar individuals often create in a flurry of hypomania or mania. Conversely, and for myself, prolific moments of artistic expression come when depression and hypomania overlap. When I'm writing, it feels as though I can do nothing else, and despite the productivity the bottom is close enough to touch. Sometimes the greatest art is the most tragic and too often the artist comes to a tragic end. Dr. Redfield Jamison continues, "That such a final, tragic, and awful thing as suicide can exist in the midst of remarkable beauty is one of the vastly contradictory and paradoxical aspects of life and art."

I don't want to romanticize this at all. When the story of the mad genius is glamorized, self-destructive behavior is often ignored, overlooked, excused, and at worst encouraged because it makes lots of money. The headline reads: "Amy Winehouse Found Dead Age 27 in London Home."

For me, my most creative contributions to life have been when I can feel death. I've climbed, made pictures, written, and spoken from this place or its scars. At times it's felt as though the creative eruption is an attempt to give the darkness light. At others it's felt as though I'm tying up loose ends before closing up shop forever.

The danger of the story of the mad genius often ends in people not seeking help because they believe it will diminish their creativity. But it's important to ask these questions: Is creation amidst destruction more valuable than life? Can balance and genius coexist, or are art and balance mutually exclusive?

Eventually, when the pain usurps the art, I'll see the fallacy of the tortured artist trope. It's a romantic identity created by culture and adopted by the individual. There is madness and there is genius and often they overlap. Pain is inevitable but suffering eventually becomes a choice. Torture isn't essential for creation no matter how sexy Hollywood makes it look.

Maybe my art comes from the confusion that something as beautiful as life can hurt so much one day and fill me with joy the next. Maybe the bipolar temperament's ability to touch those extremes is where the link lies, outside of science and explanation.

It's day twenty-eight. The skin of my face is tight from sunburn and my hair is more blond. I feel renewed and exhausted at the same time as I enter the squat medical building for the last time. I look at the shelves of disorganized pills and wonder who takes what and why. Maybe all of them could be thrown away if we all had perfect parents and siblings and no one had creepy uncles and priests.

A piece of me wants to stay here, surrounded by people who understand. My deepest self knows that sobriety isn't my forever game and I might never figure out my relationship to sex and love and all my other little vices. But at this moment I'm full of conviction. I've traded the chemicals for a new identity.

The zoo gate buzzes and I walk back into the world, sober for now.

I land back in Montana on December 24. It's blue and cold and the pine forests appear as a thick black patchwork from above. My managers, Dre and Malou, pick me up at the airport and we drive home in quiet.

I've spent most of my life seeking an instant when my frenetic mind will calm and the thoughts will order themselves and all the discontent and discomfort will drain out like dirty bathwater. It's common to misinterpret seismic shifts as singular moments that "changed everything." But this is a disservice. What we're describing is a tipping point preceded by a million moments of slow evolution, like dinosaurs sprouting feathers until they took flight and were offered a new perspective. But it's a frustrating process and sometimes we get stuck. Just ask an ostrich.

With repeated effort, we do wake up a little different every day until hindsight reveals that we are, in fact, flying. That's the nature of mindfulness and therapy and processes like CBT—tiny deliberate moments that lead to encompassing change. Profundity isn't flight but the evolution toward it. Waking up every day is profound. It's seeing moments of magic when they're offered and following them with abandon. I won't instantaneously stop smoking and drinking and fucking my way through life. And somewhere deep down I know this. But the idea that I can change the stories that drive me is a flickering lightbulb in the basement of me.

The story of being an addict is a heavy burden. It can keep us chained to our trauma. In *Chasing the Scream*, Johann Hari writes, "Addiction is an adaptation. It's not you—it's the cage you live in." It's a hopeful and powerful reprieve. Changing ourselves from the ground up by challenging and reimaging our core beliefs is the key to the cage.

The glass doors are throwing warm light onto my deck as I walk in and brush the snow from my shoes. It smells like pine because Dre and Malou have decorated a small Christmas tree tucked in the corner. The house is silent again and I fall asleep on the couch with all the lights on, still afraid of the dark.

27

These mountains that you are carrying,

you were only supposed to climb.

—Najwa Zebian

'm six months sober and it's been exactly a year since my Everest summit. The same vapors fill the same tent perched in the same spot and the same summit looms in darkness outside. I wonder if it's the same rock that has been jabbing my left ass cheek all night. Adrian has returned to Everest with a vendetta and I promised to come back here with him and we're trending on Snapchat again with the same messy hair.

Just before midnight, Adrian and a talented young Ecuadorian climber named Esteban "Topo" Mena crawl from the tent. Topo climbed Everest without oxygen when he was only twenty-three but tonight he straps a regulator to his face and turns on a steady flow and his inhalations sound like Darth Vader. He's here to support Adrian and me.

The world outside is covered in white dust that sparkles in the headlamps and the stars are obscured by clouds. I wait in the tent as the string of lights disappears into the mist and everything falls silent again. I'm waiting because history tells us that I'll be moving faster than the others and the idea is to catch them just below the summit. It's not that I'm a better athlete—Adrian has always been more fit. My only advantage is a genetic gift that allows my physiology to adapt to altitude more efficiently. Everyone's body and mind will eventually die above 26,000 feet. Mine merely dies slower.

A few hours later, I leave the tent alone and step into the familiar rhythm of my breath. Altitude does strange things to the body and my groin throbs while I worry about having testicular cancer to pass the time. I'm in the clouds and the sounds are soft and shallow. The mountain feels big, lonely, and a bit claustrophobic. My crampons scrape across stone and squeak against the cold snow while I step over the same dead bodies in tangles of rope, hanging upside down and hidden behind hoods. The equipment hanging from my harness clanks and rattles and I forget about time, listening to the team on the radio and thinking they feel far away.

When I finally see the others just after sunrise, Adrian's lips are blue and his speech is languid. But his brain is clear and he feels strong. I don't. My lethargy isn't physical fatigue. Truthfully, I'm just bored. Whatever flame had pushed me up the final 1,000 feet last year is gone. By the time I catch up, I've already decided to turn around.

I sit with Adrian as a string of climbers scrapes through the feature known as the Third Step, a small cliff band that guards the summit pyramid. We're at 28,580 feet, higher than the summit of K2. My head is loose on my neck and I feel the cold snow beneath my butt.

"Stick, I think I'm out."

"Are you sure?" He chews on candy and doesn't look up.

I pause for another moment before answering. "Yeah."

I radio base camp and tell the social media universe that I'm descending. Adrian needs to keep moving to stay warm and I wish him luck, hugging him hard with one clumsy mitten on the back of his neck. Conversations this high, in these places, take effort and have a habit of being the last words people speak. It's important to say what you mean and mean what you say, communicating as much as you can with as few words as possible. I try to catch his eyes through his reflective goggles. I know that all he can see is himself reflected back in my lenses when I say, "I love you." I mean what I say.

I say these three words a lot and have been told that the frequency diminishes the impact. Fuck that. I disagree and say them all the same, more often to men than women, and I've noticed the more they're spoken, the more they're repeated back. They're strengthened when said in truth and I can never say them too much but also understand that Love can mean a thousand different things. Adrian says, "I love you too" and I see myself staring back from his goggles. He turns up and I turn down.

I stare at the snow packed into the zippers of my boots and listen to the radios and breath of everyone on top of the world. I wait to descend crowded ropes as if I've sat down on a curb to listen to birds. It all seems so bizarre.

I don't know how long I'm sitting because time is a bit blurry here.

"Cory, what are you doing?"

I look up and see my friend Panuru Sherpa descending with a guided team.

"I think I go down," I say. "Today, I don't have." I speak in a truncated, simple way because I'm short of breath.

"But is so close!" He pulls up his goggles and smiles.

"I know. I'm tired."

"We give you oxygen and you climb. It will be good to go with Adrian."

I haven't considered putting on oxygen, because until now it wasn't an option.

"We have extra and mask."

I hesitate for a moment while he sifts through his backpack. Within a minute, there's a cylinder of oxygen tied to my back and

Panuru is saying, "Go!" Oxygen doesn't resolve the boredom, but it can lift the malaise of hypoxia. Honestly, it all happens so fast that it feels like Panuru is making the decision for me. It's a gift and I'll always be grateful.

Three hours later, I'm sitting with Adrian, Dorje Sherpa, Palden Sherpa, and Topo. Palden is much taller than me, so I'm not the highest point on the planet this year. Adrian speaks from his chest and coughs as punctuation, and the ends of his sentences seem to blow away. I've never viewed the summit as a place for celebration but rather think of it as the apex of exposure, because here I'm as far out as I can get, spent and exhausted with half the climb still ahead. If you give too much on the way up, you're more likely to blow it on the way down. I know that 61.1 percent of fatal falls in high-altitude mountaineering happen on the descent and I think of Steve Swenson telling me to "finish every climb with 10 percent left."

I hug the team and descend ahead of them and reach Camp 3 in two hours. After the summit, everything has to be removed from the mountain. I know Adrian will be exhausted by the time he gets here and he'll have little energy left to help. I stuff as much as I can to offset the burden of the others and feel selfish for going down alone. Four hours later I'm in base camp and the mountain has disappeared into thick clouds. All I can do now is sit with Monica and listen to the progress.

Four more hours pass and I see the circles of their headlamps stumbling and bobbing as little rocks shift under their feet. When he arrives, Adrian falls more than sits as the team surrounds him and gives him bent-over, awkward hugs because standing is too much now. Snow is packed in every crease and zipper and Velcro patch of his down suit. His eyes are big and severe and shell-shocked as if he's staring back up at the summit in disbelief. His cheeks are sunken and taut and his lips are swollen. His nose is burned and dark from sun. I take a picture.

It's morning now and the mountain is getting battered by heavy winds as we listen to the radio traffic of the teams still up high. Our movements are slow and achy as Adrian and I take calls and do interviews. It's his turn to shine and I like seeing him glow. This is where Adrian is his best. Climbing is his first love and that's something I can no longer claim and I think about matter changing form again. This year #EverestNoFilter will get 1.5 billion media impressions but it doesn't feel validating in the same way.

I need a media break from the noise of it all and stand outside holding a cup of hot water that tastes like metal. I think of Mom, who loves hot water with lemon. Some lemon would be good now.

Topo has dark olive skin and is boyish and handsome and speaks with a thick Ecuadorian accent. He wears black-framed glasses over narrow, dark eyes that make him look smart. His tent is filled with books and he laughs a lot, which has given him deep smile lines for his age. He's quietly magnetic and asks for no attention but is gracious when it's offered. I will never hear anyone say anything bad about him. He has his own tortures but mostly he's a person who's faced his demons and has been rewarded with humility, confidence, and joy.

I sip my water as he stands next to me and we look up at the broad northeast face of Everest and study a narrow, never-climbed couloir that intersects the ridge in the sharp black towers called the Pinnacles. Two of the best climbers in the world, Peter Boardman and Joe Tasker, vanished in the rocks in 1982. Like the line itself, their death is one of many unsolved mysteries of the Himalaya, and I picture them nestled somewhere on the ridge. I see them clearly in a faded red tent, like they went to bed and forgot to wake up.

Topo and I stand quietly. He drinks coffee and I know what he's thinking because I'm thinking it too. A new route on Everest is one of the most audacious goals in climbing and happens only once in a generation, if at all. Even imagining it takes a deliberate disregard of probability, reality, and safety. "I'd like to try to climb that."

"Me too," Topo agrees. Today we are young and confident with big imaginations and short memories and in two brief sentences the next four years of our lives are decided.

A quiet piece of me knows something I can't name because a bigger piece of me isn't ready to let go. Ninety-nine percent of me wants the massive face above us. But I haven't bothered to ask what the other 1 percent needs. To do what we're suggesting requires 100 percent, and even then there's no guarantee of survival, let alone success. A piece of me knows I'm changing form but I fear what that means.

28

The struggle itself towards the heights is enough to fill a

man's heart. One must imagine Sisyphus happy.

—Albert Camus

When the end came for him, Sisyphus, the wicked king of Corinth, escaped his demise by tricking the god of death and ensnaring him in his own chains. Later, when he found himself in Tartarus, a hellish corner of the underworld, Sisyphus cheated death again by persuading Persephone that he had been sent there by accident.

Eventually the gods caught up with him and in a way granted him his wish and allowed him to escape death forever. For his deceptions, he was sentenced for eternity to push a boulder up a mountain only to have it roll back down as he neared the summit. The real punishment of Sisyphus was eternal hopelessness.

It's May 2019 and Topo and I are standing in the same place in advance base camp, looking up at the climb. Over the past two years we've spent countless hours training, visualizing, and climbing together to bring us to this moment. In eight long hours we'll leave base camp with no oxygen and barely enough food and fuel for five days on the mountain. Above 8,000 meters, the body can burn as much as 10,000 calories a day. We are carrying 3,500 calories for every twenty-four hours. It's all we can fit in our packs; any more would make us too heavy, too slow, and all but certain to fail.

We go to bed early but I don't sleep. I never do before a climb.

I roll in my sleeping bag reading *The Obstacle Is the Way* by Ryan Holiday. The Stoic-inspired words are wise enough, telling me to "focus on the moment, not the monsters that may or may not be up ahead." In one way, climbing has been a decades-long meditation on mortality and I'm very tired. Deep in my bones, soul tired. Fear is exhausting work and has always been my greatest obstacle. It obscures the moment and paralyzes us until the moment itself has passed. Finally, my alarm goes off.

The moon is bright and I hear Topo in his tent and know that he's hopeful. I know that at some moment in the next days, I too will resign myself to hope because once you're "in it," fear is useless. Fear lives in anticipation. Hope lives in action. When the shift takes place, I will feel the joy that only climbing gives because it has never been just one thing. I need the fear for the hope for the joy and I pull on my big yellow space suit for the last time.

Goal-setting is a healthy part of life. It's deeply bound to purpose, and confronting fear and choosing hope are healthy expressions of ego. My desire to climb Everest by an unclimbed route without oxygen has very little to do with athletics. It's an act of reduction that demands everything of me without any excess. Less is more. It's a goal that requires unrealistic hope and, for me, equally heightened fear. By now I've learned that amplified risk precipitates magnified reward.

Even before they first experience symptoms, bipolar individuals tend to set higher goals and demand more of themselves. They drive harder and longer and endure more toward those ends. For many people with bipolar, there's an amplified relationship between self-worth and observable, external success. The more extreme the achievement, the more value it holds.

When an already lofty goal is achieved, the next yardstick will exceed it, exposing a susceptible mind to a potentially devastating failure. Failure is inevitable, but when identity relies on external validation, failure challenges the deepest sense of being. If we matter when we achieve, we must not matter when we fail, or so the all-or-nothing mind tells us.

In the bipolar brain, there is a strong relationship between the benchmarks of high achievement and self-worth. They are the bedrock upon which self-value is measured and identity is built. It's not a simple question of ego and this isn't your garden-variety perfectionism. Over time, perfection and self-worth and identity weave themselves together like a tree that has grown through a temple. It's no longer ornamental but structural.

Topo and I traverse the broad, flat glacier as the face begins to swallow the horizon. The snow glows neon pink and our packs feel heavy. We call these days "high gravity" and climb through the soft snow until the face is too steep to hold it, exposing the bulletproof ice underneath. Like seven years ago with Conrad, we climb unroped over terrain that is too steep to walk but not steep enough to climb. Our calves cramp and our backs ache from being too bent as we sweat out all our hydration because there's no place to stop.

We traverse right to a snow patch, but it feels hollow and likely to avalanche. Then we traverse left for 600 feet into a shallow gully where the snow is deep and slow. Topo breaks trail and our crampons slip on the ice underneath. The sun disappears over the ridge and I watch the shadow of the mountain chase our tracks 3,000 feet up the face.

I follow his steps until the shadow catches up. We've been climbing for twelve hours and have not made the progress we'd hoped. There's no place to pitch the tent because the snow only gives way to steep limestone underneath.

"What do you think?" I ask.

"It's the best we're going to get."

After an hour we've stomped out two shallow ledges just wide enough to sit but not long enough to lie down. We're tethered to the face by two small spikes of metal hammered into tiny cracks and I try not to put too much of my weight on them as I lean back and stare up. Our plan is to rehydrate and rest until dark when it's not so hot. I blink and it's dark and we're climbing again. We are two tiny dots on a black expanse of untouched, unexplored earth at 25,000 feet.

The climbing is awkward in the dark and the terrain is steeper now. I hear our crampons scrape and slip on the stone underneath. Small, falling rocks whisper by like bullets. I yell to Topo that it feels like we're getting a bit exposed and we need to wait out the darkness.

He agrees and an hour later we're back on the small snow ledges sitting in thin sleeping bags with all of our layers on. The sun will not rise for ten hours.

At 11 P.M. I'm trying to lie on my side.

At midnight I'm sitting.

It's 1 A.M. now and little sluffs of snow are pouring down on us and Topo says, "You asleep?" and I laugh and say, "Totally. Deep asleep. I really hope I wake up soon because I'm a little cold," and he laughs.

At 2 A.M. the night feels endless. "You asleep?" I chatter.

"Yes. I'm eating a hamburger."

"I'd kill a puppy for a hamburger. Can I have some?"

"Of course!" We both want to sleep. Rest would be great, but really, we just want to make the time pass. It's cold. Very, very cold.

Now it's 4 A.M. and I'm standing and kicking the stone and swinging my arms to get blood back into my fingers and toes and Topo says, "You asleep?"

"Fuuuuuuuuuck." I sit back down and look at my watch: 4:07.

Five o'clock comes and we're laughing again but I can't tell if anything is actually funny.

At six I'm begging the sun to come up and thinking that the rotation of the earth must have slowed down. There are still stars overhead, but the horizon is bright white.

At eight the sun comes and I think this night is one of the longest of my life. The light feels precious as the shadows crawl back down the mountain. When you wake up on the other side of fear, it's hope that warms you. The worst moments suddenly become the most endearing, binding you to whoever shared the burden. I start the stove, feeling more bound to Topo than any person ever.

Three hours later we've climbed another 1,000 feet, but the dark stone of the pinnacles has disappeared into the clouds and we can hear heavy wind tearing over the ridge like the constant roar of an airplane. I break trail but am exhausted from the night. I can feel that Topo has more energy and know that, despite being a decade younger than me, he's the better climber. I feel something deeper too, but it isn't fear.

Talent doesn't care how old you are. Experience does. Experience is telling me that we don't have this. Experience is telling me that this is not our time because no amount of preparation can be exchanged for timing. Experience is telling me that it's time to go down. Better sense can be heartbreaking.

The conversation is short and I can tell Topo is angry and

disappointed. He also understands this is a dangerous game and we're playing at a high level. I'm angry at me too but far less gracious toward myself because I'm not sure I entirely understand. I know we have to turn around but am confused by the calm simplicity of the moment. There is no raging storm and nothing feels dangerous. Intuition is knowing without knowing why.

We sit in the snow and suck on hard candies that have 25 calories and 4 grams of sugar each. A Snickers bar has 250 calories, 4.5 grams of fat, 33 grams of carbohydrates, 27 grams of sugar, and 4 grams of protein. I rehearse the numbers and do math and think of Dad like I always do. Dad, who taught me to sleep on ledges because these are the things one must know when climbing mountains. It's calm here, but the wind above is louder than the sun is warm and I know that whether we go up or down, gravity will win. Today it's best to work with it rather than against it.

We start downclimbing in silence, reversing our steps as the cloud ceiling drops to meet us and all the shadows and texture disappear into flat white light. The wind gets louder and chases us down as we rappel over patches of gray ice and rocks whiz by and now it's snowing. Now we're traversing back across a glacial bench and most of our tracks have been blown over and the crevasses are hard to see. Finally we're at the bottom of the face and the wind has caught up and everything is gray and cold. Topo kneels over his pack and I say, "You asleep?" He laughs but I can tell he's annoyed. Countless hours training and sweating and thinking. A thousand daydreams. Months studying pictures and theorizing. Thousands of dollars. All of this, two years of effort, for two days of climbing.

We've all heard that the summit doesn't matter but right now I think that might be something said to make us feel better about not getting there. It certainly doesn't make me feel any better back in base camp while I pack my bags and wipe crumbs and old pieces of floss from the corners of my empty tent. The summit doesn't matter. But then again, it kind of does. The summit matters because it's the source of hope itself. It's what brings us to the process to begin with. Only the view from the summit can illuminate its own insignificance.

There's a piece of me that knows I'm done climbing and that this has nothing to do with worth or value. I've sacrificed joy for unreasonable expectations of myself. Because it's the apex of the planet, I've always understood Everest as unifying. I choose to see it as the singular point from which all else flows, outward and downward, its slopes continuing beyond the base of the mountain and wrapping the world together. That's a pretty impossible thing to measure your worth against.

I hear the rocks crunch under my feet and feel entirely drained as Topo and I walk away from the mountain. The yak bells are clanging and the ice is melting and the Tibetans are whistling and I'm breathing thicker and thicker air. I'm scared of not living up to my own story and am still hopeful that I can push the boulder over the hill. I don't imagine Sisyphus as happy. I imagine him as hopeful. Topo walks behind me and I say, "Next year?" over my shoulder.

"Yes, of course! But first, a hamburger."

III

29

When I pronounce the word Future,

the first syllable already belongs to the past.

—Wislawa Szymborska

'm nine years old and open the door of the rusty blue Suburban that always smells like wet dog. The door squeaks and slams loudly because there's just a track of glue around the edges where the rubber used to be. Dad climbs onto the other side of the bench seat and positions a piece of plywood behind his lower back to ease the pain of a disc that slipped out of place when he was remodeling the upstairs bathroom and tried to lift a bathtub on his own. Because that is what fathers do.

On most car rides, he tunes the radio to NPR, which seems to make the car hotter and the smell of dogs more pungent. But today he loads a Paul Simon cassette and the car swallows it with a series of plastic clicks. I roll down the window and imagine this is the soundtrack of my life while playing with the late summer air in a cupped hand that rises and falls like a wave.

My arm hairs vibrate in the wind and I wonder when my hands will look strong and vascular like Dad's as he grips the worn-smooth steering wheel with one and drinks coffee from a cheap plastic mug with the other. He belts out the lyrics and hums when he doesn't know the words. This summer he has a thick sandy beard that almost hides the dark red mole on his right cheek. When there are no lyrics, he whistles and taps his fingers against the steering wheel. To me he's perfect because he has sun wrinkles that make him look like he's just come down from a mountain and his eyes have trapped the sky.

The roads of Salt Lake City spread out from the Mormon temple as numbered blocks in four directions: 500 East, 1200 South. But to me, all numbers remind me of Dad because above all things he loves numbers. He loves them alongside Mom and my brother and me because, unlike the three of us, he can always make sense of them. In numbers he can prove that despite the asymmetries and disorder of life, underlying it all is an elegant and unshakable mathematical bedrock. This is why he teaches math to teenagers. Because everyone needs to know that there is something reliable in the world, especially when the world seems so unreliable.

We park in an empty parking lot and I notice the minerals of cheap asphalt catching rays and sparkling. It's another of the sun's many tricks, throwing light in ways that can make ugly things beautiful.

When no one is looking, I still hold Dad's hand. When anyone is looking, I puff out my chest and turn away and pretend that it was never him who put Band-Aids on my knees and wiped my ass long after I should've stopped shitting my pants. But no one here is looking and I'm an extension of him as our shadows merge into one: a unified but terribly lopsided m wobbling over the asphalt. In mathematics, m represents the rate of change.

The building rises in hard right angles and looks just like the streets, only tipped on its side. Dad says it's 90°, but I confuse angles and temperature and say it must be at least 105°.

"A hundred and five degrees?" he says incredulously.

"At *least*!" I'm very certain of many things.

"I don't know . . . looks like 90° to me." He has an upper hand in a game I don't know we're playing because that's what fathers do. They fuck with you. They make you more and less certain of everything and you hope they do it with love instead of fists. I am one of the lucky ones who never knows a father's hands as anything other than tools of creation and care.

I drop his callused palm and enter the drab building to a blast of cool air, rushing into a world of math and art and the place where our minds can communicate. On a maze of walls hang lithographs, woodblocks, sketches, and tessellations of impossible symmetry. Dad isn't a connoisseur of modern art but he can't resist the mathematical genius of M. C. Escher.

The tessellations are his favorite, especially the one called *Day and Night*, where the negative space of white geese becomes black geese flying in the opposite direction. The white flock fly into a night sky, the black into day.

But I don't have time for the subtlety of the designs and am transfixed by a dragon twisted into an infinite knot, eating its own tail because it's mysterious and confusing. It's called an ouroboros.

"Which one is your favorite?" he asks.

"I can't decide. But I like this one."

"Hmmmph," he says, more as a question than a statement, and I wonder if I should change my mind.

"Which one is yours?" I ask.

"I like this one," he says, pointing at the geese, and tries to describe why it is so mathematically special.

"I like that one too." I want to be like him.

"Why?"

"I don't know."

"You don't know why you like it?"

"I just think it's cool."

"Yeah, it's *cool*."

After some more highly intellectual art critique, we both settle in front of a lithograph called *Drawing Hands* in which two hands draw each other in a repeating cycle of creation from nothing. The hands remind me of Dad's when he does impossibly long equations that look like he's forgotten that numbers and letters are different. The hands have less hair than his but the same strong veins. This drawing is its own echoing of an ouroboros.

The oldest known ouroboros was found on the Golden Shrine in King Tut's tomb, representing the infinite nature of time as it flows back into itself. Specific to Egypt, it represented the cycles of the Nile and the sun's daily descent into the waters of Nun, where it braved a primeval void full of cosmic obstructions until rising again into an unencumbered sky. The symbol and its meaning are ubiquitous in art, belief, and philosophy, always representing the nature of time, destruction, death, rebirth, and the interconnectedness of all things. But for now all I see are Dad's hands that do math, lift bathtubs, hold coffee cups, tap their fingers to Paul Simon, and sweep infinite amounts of dog hair from the car even though it always smells the same.

While Dad stands in front of a drawing of stairs that somehow climb up and down at the same time, I sneak away to the gift shop and use twenty dollars Mom gave me to buy him a tie for his birthday. This one has a delicate tessellation of red and navy geese flying in opposite directions, so it's perfect for him even though he doesn't wear ties and has no use for gifts.

Twenty-nine years later, I wonder how many kids bought ties for fathers who were forced to wear them by conscientious mothers, who were aware that their children wanted to know Dad loved them. This occurs to me in a teahouse on the border of Nepal and Tibet when Mom calls and tells me that Dad has terminal liver cancer.

I think about the serpent eating its tail and hands drawing themselves and begin to understand the ouroboros.

The morning after the call I wake before dawn on a plywood bed in a room with a packed dirt floor. The thick scent of burning yak dung and juniper slides under the door and settles against the walls. Ten years ago I woke up in the same village to the same smells. I wonder if the same yaks are still alive, their waste becoming the fuel for the fire keeping me warm and heating the salty butter tea that's steaming up the kitchen. A strong breeze is rattling the single-pane windows that don't close all the way. Ten years ago I was photographing my first assignment for the magazine. Ten years ago I was filled with angst and anticipation and fire. I was engaged and in love. I was a climber. I was a photographer. My father's liver was healthy and I was still very certain of many things.

But this morning I'm certain of less and wander outside, tiptoeing up the stairs that bend and creak no matter where I step or how light I imagine myself to be. They're painted a glossy brown that appears black and the wood railing feels rough in my hand. From the second floor I climb a stepped log to the dirt roof where the wind is strong, spilling off the Tibetan Plateau and funneling through the towering gorge of the Kali Gandaki River.

On the roof, I light a cigarette called a Surya Luxury King. In America, I call them Marlboro Lights. I've smoked many cigarettes with many different names and I wish I'd quit because now cancer is real. But this morning the wind is blue and cold and the ember glows pink and orange and offers me a moment to think about Dad and the assignment and Dad and the pictures I need to make and Dad.

An hour later the sun spills into the gorge as the jeep jumps back in time ten years, driving under the caves where Lincoln's head exploded and where there was no road but now there is because everything is changing. The road is the reason I'm back

in the same place that I started my career for *National Geographic,*
where I'll end my career for *National Geographic.*

When Mustang opened its gates to tourism in 1992, at about
the same time I was looking at M. C. Escher drawings with Dad,
the kingdom was connected by ancient trails sneaking south
off the Tibetan Plateau. Eventually the paths funneled into a
braided network that followed the river basin, creating the most
direct path from China to India as an offshoot of the Silk Road.
The trails were worn by centuries of foot traffic and trade cara-
vans that flooded the kingdom with wealth from the fourteenth
century onward. But in 2008 the monarchy of Mustang was absorbed by the politics of Kathmandu. At the same time, China
was helping consolidate the trails into a rough-hewn through-
way, part of a larger project, aptly named the New Silk Road, that
would connect the ancient kingdom to Beijing and Delhi. With
new economic and political forces sculpting the landscape, the
space for a king was erased and Jigme Singhi Palbar Bista, a direct descendant of Ame Pal, the first king of Mustang, became
suspended between past and present. To Mustangis he is still a
king, connected to the outside world by a road that both aids and
destroys the people he serves.

I think of Jigme's predicament and how much has changed in
the past decade. The first time I came here, I walked. The second
time, I rode a horse. The third time, I bounced in the back of an
enormous truck that looked like the skeleton of a Transformer, a
cage around the bed circling over me like steel ribs. I spread out
over a heap of duffels and let the Himalayan sun darken my
freckles. But even then there was no real road, just pieces of one
that forced the convoys into the mouth of a steep slot canyon to
navigate the bends of the river. Now the relative comfort of the
old Land Cruiser seems luxurious as the vehicle winds its way up
a single lane through blown-out sandstone cliffs that fall away
thousands of feet to the riverbed where the big trucks used to
drive.

My childhood was filled with roads like this and I remember Dad driving the Burr Trail through the Utah desert, winding our way down washed-out hairpin turns between sandstone monoliths while Paul Simon serenaded the family.

Dad always drove and I always trusted his hands and instead watched Mom as she gripped the "oh shit" handle, inhaling terse sips of oxygen that helped her brace against inevitable doom. I watched the tendons in her wrist pop out and understood that my arms and hands would never look like his but instead would resemble hers. Delicate. Sinewy. Strong. When the road finally flattened, she'd exhale long and deep and say "Wooooo" in a tone that straddled annoyance and relief and then turn to tickle my feet.

I see them in flashbacks as I drive further into the landscape, putting in earbuds and listening to my family soundtrack. It feels like everything here is trying to tell me something: "It was a dry wind and it swept across the desert and it curled into the circle of birth / And the dead sand falling on the children / The mothers and the fathers of the automatic earth."

After eight hours, the jeeps dip into the shadows of the mountains and grind their way toward an enclave of earthen homes, goat pens, and orchards. The village sits in a small depression with willow, sour apple, and wild olive trees. It appears as an oasis suspended in the fifteenth century, when kings were still kings. Whitewashed mud construction is splashed with burnt orange and gray, the colors of the Sakya sect of Buddhism reminding me, as everything here does, that nothing is forever.

In the morning, I traverse the broken terraces of one of the king's palaces that's fallen into disrepair. Grass, seeds, and small stones crumble from the cracks of broken walls that are no longer level. Some lean precariously over the eroding cliff falling away to the river below. The foundational wall leans at least 105° and I remember Dad saying 90° and I laugh because after twenty-nine years I finally get the joke.

In a damp grove of yellowing willows, a baby yak stands tethered to a pole chewing on a pile of grass, staring curiously as I climb a ladder onto a dirt roof. Kyle, Ben, Lisa, and Tsewang, the first cousin of the king, lift the lights and cameras and pass them between dirty hands with dust in the wrinkles of their knuckles. Because even if there was a hot shower, the soil of Mustang never washes away. Once you've crawled up the ladders, heard the yak bells and the guttural barks of Tibetan mastiffs, and smelled the acrid burning dung and juniper, once you've heard drums and horns that crawl over the monastery walls, you simply don't want to wash it off because the dirt under your nails makes you a part of it.

A handsome novice monk leads us gleefully through the decaying rooms with shafts of sunlight shooting through dusty air. He jumps over a dark hole in the floor and I watch loose rubble fall in and make a crackling noise as it hits an invisible bottom. And there is cancer again, eating my dad's liver. I've always seen the world in metaphor, but now it's everywhere and in everything. Cancer is as insidious in the minds of loved ones as it is in the body it's killing.

Tsewang unravels a chain, unlocks a padlock, and pushes open the door, which squeaks like the Suburban. The room is dusty and our feet leave scuffed footprints and kick up the floor in silent gray puffs. Pillars prop up the low ceiling and a dirty window floods the room with a soft yellow glow. It smells dense and old with hints of decaying wood and forgotten things. A broom and dustpan rest bored in the corner until our monk chaperone begins to sweep the sand.

Stacked against another wall is a collection of treasures that reach back to the first king of Mustang. Sculptures and paintings and statues from the fifteenth century stare at us and I wonder if the effigies are happy to have company. Because to Buddhists these are not just things but living gods with real life inside of them. I wonder how long it's been since they've had visitors and if they get bored and talk to the broom and dustpan that make the dirt floor clean.

I go about the business of setting up the lights and tripod and positioning the relics. Sculpted faces of ancestors and gods are dotted with real gems and auspicious stones laid in ornate crowns. Tattered pages of monastic books and histories are decorated with delicate, eight-hundred-year-old paintings of Buddha and monsters and tigers. On the adjacent wall swords and clubs from ancient battles hang alongside morbid masks with bright, wide eyes and sharp teeth. Amidst the collection hangs a mummified human hand of "the last person who stole from the king."

Art is a vessel of history and the physical manifestation of story. It holds the beliefs and understanding of ourselves and where we've come from in a way that no other thing can. It anchors us to the stories of the past that are essential to our future. It's a reduction that distills and holds the most vital elements of culture and offers them back when we begin to forget. It's also incredibly valuable. As in dollars and cents.

As the road from China is completed, more and more ancient art disappears from rooms just like this. Hungry traders, collectors, and tourists drive the road and stop in the villages and offer enormous piles of cash to families who have none. The sale of even a small statue from the twelfth or thirteenth century can pay for an entire college education for multiple children. But once the child moves to Kathmandu or New York or Berlin, they rarely come back. And if something isn't for sale, it often goes missing anyway. I understand that there's a difference between something being stolen and something being bought. The people who take the relics home aren't necessarily "stealing," so their hands won't end up mummified on a wall. Either way, something leaves and never comes back.

I carefully place the lights to cast dramatic shadows across the pile of relics, take a photo, and wonder how much they're worth. I take a portrait of the string of swords that protected the kingdom against invaders but are of no use against a road. I capture an image of the novice monk holding a tattered painting as he looks through the yellow window and into an uncertain future.

Two days later, just after 9 A.M., a Buddhist holy man arrives on a brown mule. He's wearing a filthy yellow golf shirt and I guess his age at somewhere between seventy-five and three hundred years old.

After rolling out a small rug, he throws a red monastery pillow on the ground and creaks to his knees. His fingers wade through loose monastic texts as he licks his cracked lips and stares through Coke-bottle glasses so scratched I can't imagine they help him see at all. Finally he settles on a page and the rumbling voice of a much younger man spills out, chanting from a guttural place deep in his stomach. His eyes follow Tibetan calligraphy across yellowed pages, pausing occasionally to clear phlegm and pour raksi, a local rice wine that tastes like sake and vodka. He decants some into a wooden teacup and drinks it. He pours another serving into a simple chalice made from the top of a human skull, adorned on the rim by small pinches of dirty butter, emptying the milky fluid from a large plastic Coke bottle because everything here is old and new at the same time.

To his left I watch a shirtless Loba man with a white bandana over his nose and mouth swing an axe and my brain struggles to interpret what I'm witnessing. Each blow lands with a wet thud, cutting through lifeless human flesh and breaking bone, sending small pieces of wet skin and muscle and watery blood splattering. Of all the dead bodies I've witnessed in life, I've never seen anything quite like this.

Sky burials are the charnel practice of excarnation, where the deceased is disemboweled and laid out to decompose and be scavenged, most often by enormous Himalayan vultures. Because Tibetan Buddhism believes in the transmigration of spirits, the body of the dead is an empty vessel and of no importance because the soul has closed up shop and moved on. To the outside world, it appears barbaric. But to the people of Mustang and much of Central Asia, it's both symbolic and practical. A sky burial is the Buddhist's last act of compassion, feeding an expired physical form back into the living world. To witness the practice is to watch the snake eating its tail.

The body is little more than cyan skin stretched over a skeleton threatening to push through the flesh. Before the axes, it was stripped naked and laid out like an X. Two men removed their shoes and shirts and pragmatically went to work scalping the head with its coarse gray hair and making a series of long incisions on the arms and legs before cutting into the belly.

The stomach cavity and organs are removed and the mess is laid over the stones. The liver is a dark purple-black and one of the men stops to inspect it before throwing it aside. It lands with the sound of a saturated rag and he returns to work and I think of Dad and wonder what his liver looks like.

I turn my camera to silent so there is no noise when I shoot.

It's hot and I'm sweating into my eyes and the sun is too bright for photography. The world appears with too much contrast, like light is pressing itself against the seams of everything. Mud cliffs rise above and watch as indifferent sentinels. They've witnessed a thousand sky burials. The caves that brought me here ten years ago serve as perches for the vultures to collect before they descend on the body to feast and I see that everything has a role in the process.

But today the birds aren't coming. The lama chants and rings a brass bell and blows through a kangling, a trumpet made from a human femur he uses to call in the vultures. *His* vultures that he knows by name and that come to all sky burials he presides over. He blows more. And still the sky is empty. The birds have been coming less and less in Mustang, driven out by deliberate poisoning and human persecution, diminishing livestock to scavenge, and a road that seems to tie it all together.

He stops blowing. The birds never come.

The men return to the body and begin stripping the flesh and throwing it in the river. They smash the bones to pieces and throw them in too. Eventually they break the skull with the back of the axe and set a small piece aside before throwing the blades of their tools in the juniper fire to purify them and wash them clean of any malign spirits that might have hung on in the process. They strip naked and dip their sinewy frames into the water and scrub themselves clean. After dressing, they return to the lama to drink the raksi and blur their vision and forget the work of chopping a body to pieces.

Back in the house of the deceased, I drink butter tea in silence as the family remembers a person in fragments who became fish food. I remember burying the body in Peru and the other bodies frozen on mountains and imagine their families piecing them together as a collection of stories.

Eventually the men who performed the preparation of the body are very drunk. The lama stands and tips too far forward on his toes and wavers the way drunk people do when they're trying to hide it. He bows gently and offers the piece of skull to the daughter, who will burn it to ash, mix it with clay, and press it into tiny auspicious molds called *tsa tsa*. The effigies will be left as offerings at holy sites so that life persists after the living is done.

As I stand to leave, I notice a blood-red geometric figure painted over the door. Overlapping lines weave in and out of each other in a series of 90° angles that appear as the peaks of *m*'s and I think of my dad and mathematics and the rate of change. The symbol has no end and no beginning, feeding back into itself. This is Buddhism's ouroboros and it's called the Endless Knot.

Mustang, the reluctant king, the road and dust and tractors, my father and cancer and family, art and history and future, my career, the boy I was and the person I'm becoming and Paul Simon and the hands drawing themselves somehow are all woven together in the same unending loop.

30

What I look forward to is continued

immaturity followed by death.

—DAVE BARRY

A month later I'm sitting with Mom and Dad talking about things like radiation and transplants and chemotherapy and white blood cells and liver enzymes and something called a "count." The term *hepatocellular carcinoma* is discussed, and I forget it immediately because I don't believe it. They call it HCC, which is a medical term for "your liver is fucked."

Mom and I talk about Dad as if he isn't sitting just a few feet from us.

"Well, he's very tired," she says.

"Can he get a transplant?"

"Dad doesn't have enough healthy liver left to attach a new one to. Besides, he's too old."

"Yeah, he is old as fuck. We should probably get moving on your Tinder profile." We laugh because there's nothing else to do. Dad leans back and looks at the floor with his reading glasses pinching the end of his nose, staring into something that we all know is there but no one can see.

One hand hangs at his side and he clicks the fingernails of his thumb and middle finger together. It sounds like a clock keeping unfair time that rushes and drops seconds. Mom keeps talking and he keeps nodding without breaking his stare.

"So how much time is there?" I ask.

"Generally, eleven months."

"Do we know when eleven months started?" I wonder how long he's been clicking his nails like this, and someone answers, "No."

I always reach for my camera when the unthinkable happens and I want to make a film about family and dying and cancer. Telling stories of pain is a way to understand my own. Now I want to tell the story of our family before a piece of it is lost. I don't want to watch but I can't look away. I want to understand us to understand myself.

Mom and Dad agree to let the cameras into the house and I bring a team in to document, direct, produce, interview, and film walls of family pictures while my mom tells short stories. "Oh, isn't that just adorable?" she says, and points to a picture of me. I'm five years old with offensively blond hair, sitting on one of Dad's many decks. My head is pitched back, eyes closed, as I soak up sun and hold an apple. I wonder if she wishes I would've stayed trapped in that innocence forever.

I go to a radiation appointment and shove myself into a small, sterile room with wires and syringes and a bed with rails. Dad takes off his plaid shirt and jeans and places his shoes on a chair. He was never shy about nakedness growing up, but he seems more timid now, as if he's embarrassed by what time has done. He turns his back to put on a gown and I help him tie it and notice the odd shape of old men. The strong, powerful legs that I used to follow up trails have become skinny. One calf has almost disappeared since the bones in his ankle were fused together. A quadricep peeled back a few years later and never fully healed. Everything has atrophied aside from his stomach, which has grown. I can tell that his mind is still thirty-four years old, but his body has betrayed him.

Two hours later I pick him up after the doctors have run a catheter up the inside of his groin and blasted radiation on the tumors. My friend Tommy Joyce is filming while Dad finishes a club sandwich and crumples the red-and-white deli paper into a ball, tucking it in his pocket to keep my car clean.

"Are you nauseous?" I ask.

"A little, I guess."

"Okay, well, just let me know if you need me to pull over." But he's already staring out the windshield wide-eyed and before he can roll down the window no less than a gallon of carrot-colored vomit volcanoes from his nose and mouth across the dashboard and windows and down his puffy red jacket. The acid is making him cry as he retches and spits leftover chunks from his teeth. We continue home as he apologizes and fakes laughter, embarrassed. I try to comfort him by saying it's okay and normal while I struggle to hold back tears.

I spend an hour wiping radioactive pieces of turkey club from the cracks of the console, alternating between dry heaves and tears. The smell will likely never go away, but even if it does, there's footage of the entire event, so the memory never will.

For Christmas, I give Dad a T-shirt with a grim reaper holding a scythe standing ominously above the words "Just Here to Party." I give Mom perfectly ugly teacups that say "Fuck Cancer" in gold. I give Dad a card featuring the image of a headstone that says "RIP." Above the grave, it says, "I HOPE YOU DIE." Underneath where the body is buried, it says, ". . . after a really long fulfilling life because I love you so incredibly much." He laughs and then cries because there is still nothing else to do.

Dad rolls out of bed with his glasses strung around his neck because he likes to read in the morning. He uses a cane to stand and groans and chuckles because the cameras are rolling and he feels like a movie star. I photograph him in his loose underwear in the bathroom getting pills from a cabinet with more bottles than I can count. I don't want to objectify him, but all the cameras help separate me from the reality of what I'm witnessing in the same way a war photographer's cameras keep them at a distance from the horror.

Watching him die from cancer is more like watching him fade away, as if his opacity is being reduced. It's jarring and subtle at the same time, an irreconcilable disconnect between his failing body and his living mind. I don't really believe the diagnosis because he sits in front of me and tells the same jokes that I've grown to hate but now long for before the punch lines leave the air.

He calls ketchup "cat shit" and mustard "mouse turd" and sandwiches "sammies" and lets mayonnaise sit in the corners of his mouth far too long before he wipes it away. He eats vanilla ice cream with saltines on top. He loves the crunch of iceberg lettuce. He asks, "Have you seen the latest whatever climbing magazine?" because he wants to talk to me so badly. I say no, because I don't care about climbing anymore even though I'm still planning to return to Everest. Instead, I want him to say something profound to me about the meaning of life. He tries again and asks, "Did you ever read so-and-so's account of the first ascent of such-and-such on the border of somewhere?" And I say no.

The power of his voice is incongruous with his hazy physical presence. Hard edges are becoming soft, lazy lines that fade into something I can't see and I'm worried that when he finally disappears his voice will haunt me. He'll ask questions I don't have the answers to, asking for time I refused to give him when there was still time at all.

His skin is crepey and thin like tissue paper with a faint wax layer over the top and freckled by liver spots. He bruises without being touched and spontaneously bleeds on the new furniture

Mom is buying, trying to fill up the space he'll leave behind. But the tiny bloodstains won't let her forget, no matter how many couches she buys. It will be his final joke, a trail of breadcrumbs that always leads her back to their life together. He picks at a scab while she asks for my help buying a new chair. He spills his coffee on the new rug and Mom loses her mind. "Jesus fucking Christ, Courtney! This is why I can't have anything nice!" she almost cries. She's buying furniture and mistaking it for time. But everything she tries to put in the space he's leaving behind will only serve as reminders of where he no longer is. Watching him die is hard. Watching her live is excruciating.

She says, "Alexa, play Paul Simon," bending over the device and screaming as if Alexa is hard of hearing. Alexa says, "Okay, which album?"

She laughs and says, "Shit . . . I don't know."

"I'm sorry, I didn't catch that."

"Pick one."

On the last leg of a journey they started a long time ago
The arc of a love affair.

Dad and I slip out of the house and go to Sam's Brewery and I watch him drink a beer and wipe his eyes, which seem to be getting bluer by the hour. After a long pause, he says, "Your mother raised you boys." I think of my brother and wonder where he is. We barely speak aside from an occasional text on birthdays and holidays. But this isn't about us. He cries and reaches for my hand. "I did nothing. I'm sorry."

"That's not true. Look at what I do. You don't think that has something to do with you?" I wish I had more, better words. I always thought there would be so much more to say and it feels like there is but suddenly I'm mute. I also know that when he disappears from the other side of the table all the words I'm looking for will show up because death and words are always too early and too late, respectively.

He cries and I hold his hand and we become a seated *m*. For a moment the hands drawing themselves become one and the ouroboros stalls. The endless knot constricts. The roads of our lives overlap and the reluctant king of my life sips his beer and thinks about the things he still needs to say. He's lost because there are no numbers. This equation isn't mathematical. The sum of everything is infinity and the sum of infinity is 1—or maybe oneness. It's an unending loop and only one thing seems to give it any meaning at all. After a long silence he says, "I love you so much."

I park the car in the garage and watch him hobble toward the door. His pants are more air than flesh. His hair is more salt than pepper. His back is more curved than straight. And to me he is perfect because of his sun wrinkles and his eyes that just keep accumulating sky. As death approaches, it seems they have become hungrier for life.

I film his tools hanging above his workbench. I film sawdust and a coffee can of miscellaneous screws and washers and nuts. I film a tattered leather tool belt. I film skis and poles and dog collars from a lifetime of dog hair that never sweeps away. I film ice axes and ropes and dusty camping chairs. He opens the door behind me and it slams shut while the dog door swings on its hinges. "We're home!" he hollers for the two millionth time and Mom says "Hi!" and Paul Simon sings:

There may come a time when I will lose you
Lose you as I lose my sight, days falling backward into velvet night.

I can't tell whom he's singing to.

31

Imagine living in a world where there is no domination,
where females and males are not alike or even always
equal, but where a vision of mutuality is the
ethos shaping our interaction.

—BELL HOOKS

There is no easy way to write this chapter and I don't want to. There will be no consensus and not everyone will be content. It's a trigger-laden minefield. There's no way to tie it in a bow or satisfy the many opinions and ideas. I want to. I can't. Every piece of me wants to leave the page blank and forget. But this book isn't about the easy way and it isn't about omission. In this context, saying nothing changes nothing. If you aren't confused by the end of it, I haven't explained it clearly.

I don't remember what happens that night and I don't know when it occurs, but I'll be told it's 2015, before Everest and rehab and Dad's Swiss cheese liver. *What follows is not a memory.* It's a re-creation, and I imagine it happened like this:

It's January and I'm in Washington, D.C., for the annual Photographer's Seminar. I've spent four days with colleagues and friends.

Tonight, all the seriousness will be danced on, laughed out, and left on the floor.

By the time I end up at the party, I've already had a few drinks and am feeling gregarious and playful and my boundaries are blurry. The room is dark and squares of light spin from a disco ball and the quiet of the street is replaced by blended voices clawing to be heard over too-loud music. Wyclef Jean is covering the Bee Gees through the speakers, saying something about staying alive. I feel the hot, humid air of sweat and breath and too many people packed into too small a space. A group of friends and colleagues are standing in a circle and don't see me come in and I sneak up behind a woman and give a swift, surprising spank to announce my arrival and then I erase the memory forever.

That I can forget is emblematic of a larger issue.

It's May 19, 2020, and I think it's too warm for spring in Colorado as I carry an armload of groceries to my car. My phone is ringing and I feel flustered as I try to unlock the door and free up my hands before whoever is calling hangs up.

"Hello?"

A firm but pleasant woman says, "Is this Cory Richards?"

"It is. Who's this?"

She's calling from *National Geographic*. "I'm a lawyer in the human resources department and we've received an anonymous letter. Do you have time to talk?" I don't hold the steering wheel as much as push it away, twisting my hands and overgripping until my forearms hurt. "The letter contains some accusations that we're currently investigating," she continues.

One accusation is regarding a sexual joke I made in a group at a party, probably in a bar or under spinning disco lights. She repeats a punch line and I don't remember the specifics but honestly it sounds like me. Guilty.

The second accusation is the spank and I can't remember it at all as the lawyer asks, "Do you have a reputation for being flirty? I understand you like to drink and have maybe had too much at times." I'm ashamed because this is true but is no excuse.

"I haven't had a drink in four years. How long ago did this happen?"

"Five years."

"Does the letter say who I touched?"

"Yes." She gives me a name and I'm more confused.

The woman who I goosed is someone I deeply respect and trust.

"Have you asked her?"

"Yes. And she has corroborated the accusation and provided context. We're trying to understand." I have nothing to say because I'm trying to understand too and question the context she's referring to. The air-conditioning is blasting but I'm sweating and my hands feel cold. My face is flushed and she asks, "Are you still there? This is very serious."

"Yes." I pause. "If she says it happened, it happened. I trust her. Can you give me more information?"

"Not at this time."

I'm offered the option to hire an attorney, but she reminds me that it would be an escalation. I consider it for a moment but know that I have a habit of turning candles into house fires. Besides, I've already admitted that I fucked up. I don't want it to be true, but I do have offside humor and have conceded that, considering the corroboration, the allegation of an inappropriate touch must be true as well. It doesn't matter that I don't remember. That I *presumably* thought it was playfulness is not an excuse. That I didn't understand how inappropriate it was is like telling a police officer that I didn't know the speed limit or I didn't know how fast I was going. Both can be true, but it's still my responsibility to know. I also feel cornered, defensive, and defiant and use words like "absurd" and "silly."

I'm furious that the letter is anonymous. I'm angry that I can't remember and I'm frustrated that I can't simply call and apologize. I seethe because there is no defense and even if there was, there's no forum in which to offer it. I'm screaming to myself, "It was a joke!" and "How do I apologize for something I don't remember?"

The lawyer tells me that I'm to have no communication with anyone about the accusations until their investigation is complete and that discussion risks further punishment. She tells me that I've been suspended, and I know that even when this is resolved, the scar will likely never go away.

"How long do you think this is gonna take?" I ask.

"Six months," she says, but what she really means is a lifetime. It will be my responsibility to share and live with this story forever, and I will feel shame every time I have to bring it up.

I stand in my kitchen with my girlfriend, Melissa, and feel sick to my stomach, facing a woman I love and admitting to something I've never understood. Her eyes are bloodshot with tears. She wrings her hands and I see that her knuckles are white and the tendons of her wrists are tight underneath tattoos that I've always loved. She's torn between her experience with men and her love for me as she explains the full breadth of her experience as a woman, which is something I can never fully understand. Mom cries too, concerned for me, frustrated by it all, and unjustly furious with herself, and I hear her silently say, "I raised you better."

With nothing else to do, I pour all the energy and angst into training for my return to Everest with Topo, trying to sweat out confusion and anger. I spend hours in a chamber of recycling thoughts and arguments, monologuing to invisible faces about how absurd and unfair it all is. I exhaust myself day after day until I'm too tired to think. I'm sorry for the joke and I'll do better and I think it's all a little silly all at the same time because nothing is clear as I lie on my bed and stare at the ceiling.

The accusation of the spank is a clearer violation. Despite my presumed assumption of playfulness and humor, I understand why it's considered sexual even if there was nothing intentionally sexual about it. Presumption doesn't excuse it or make it less inappropriate, and I read article after article on what constitutes sexual assault. It all feels a bit gross. I do too.

I haven't showered after a long training session and I smell like an unwashed skunk. My skin is crinkly from dried salt and my feet are wrinkled from sweat. Little fibers are stuck to my toes, and I can feel tiny splashes of oil on my belly leaping up from a hot pan. As the pandemic rages and one lockdown weaves into another, my days have been reduced to training and eating and reading. Rupert, my dog, is trying to understand why he can't have chicken, and I'm trying to understand why I can't just apologize and I read an article in *The New York Times* titled "Publicly, We Say #MeToo. Privately, We Have Misgivings" by Daphne Merkin. She writes, "The fact that such unwelcome advances persist, and often in the office, is, yes, evidence of sexism and the abusive power of the patriarchy."

One of the issues is that photographers in my position have been seen as impervious in the same way actors and musicians are. They've often been wrongfully excused for inappropriate behavior because they hold an outsized degree of power. That isn't okay. In the context of power, however, I still don't totally get it. At *National Geographic,* I always understood myself as subordinate. From this perspective, as my superior, the position she held could make or break my career in an instant. But again, there's a

power dynamic that I'm responsible for regardless if I understand it or not. I read more and think it's confusing how two
people standing next to each other can experience the same relationship from opposite poles.

It's autumn now and several months have passed with no word.
I'm walking up a trail panting alongside Rupert. My muscles
ache and I notice how taut they are, stretched and stressed and
tired. I pass a man in a full space helmet breathing through an air
purifier who steps no less than nineteen feet off the trail because
everyone is on edge, isolated, and flooded with stress, afraid of
dying from the plague. I pull up my mask and try to smile with
my eyes. As I get back to the car, it starts to snow and I feel my
phone vibrate.

"Is this Cory Richards?" It's a new attorney, but I recognize
the tone and brace myself. He tells me the initial recommenda-
tion of the legal team is that *National Geographic* sever ties with
me in perpetuity because the "risk of association is too great." I've
learned a lot about all the garbage that women endure and am
becoming fluent. I drive home listening to his voice and the specifics and think about my blind spots as I unlock the door. At
least now maybe I can move on. Maybe I'll even be able to apologize.

Humor is important. Laughter and playfulness, like everything
we do, evolved to help us survive. Infants start developing humor
at six weeks, and they drool and blow bubbles and squeal. Laughter helps develop the motor cortex, frontal lobe, and limbic system and helps regulate serotonin levels. It limits stress hormones
like cortisol that damage metabolic function, the cardiovascular
system, and immune response. Because of limbic resonance, shared

humor strengthens social bonds and intimacy and draws us into community. By these measures, laughter and play are two of the body's many remedies for stress, anxiety, and depression. Studies have shown that even reading "hahaha" changes our brain chemistry.

Humor is also complex. It comes in many nuanced forms and some of them are aggressive. Passive joking is a subtle form of "truth"-telling by communicating something without actually saying or doing it. It allows us to hide behind the pretense of humor and I hear myself saying, "It was just a joke. I was playing." But now I'm whispering because I'm not so sure.

The lawyer's voice has mostly faded to background noise.

"Are you still there?"

"Yeah, Sorry. I'm listening." It hurts that it's come to this. My lingering anger is just an extension of the pain.

"*But*," he continues, "in light of the context that's been provided, as well as the people who have spoken for you, we have decided *not to* sever ties. I'm supporting that decision."

His voice is stern and my teeth are grinding and my hands are gripping because I am waiting for the bad news, but it never comes.

"Everything is concluded. I sincerely hope we never speak again."

I exhale and think that's the best way for any lawyer to hang up the phone.

But even though my name is cleared, there's no way back and I know it. Despite the fact that the situation is nuanced, my career with *National Geographic* is likely over. It's not that I can't work for them, but that the experience has irrevocably altered the psychology of all of us. For me it's too painful and embarrassing. For them it's too fresh and my place has already been filled up. In this case, it's easier for everyone just to move on.

Being investigated for over a year has been deeply troubling, difficult, and traumatic. At times, I've been furious. I've been angry at women and that's scared me. I've also thought I'm angry at feminism. There were times I believed I was a victim. The truth is, I just didn't get it at all because I've never had to.

But despite what angry men on YouTube these days are yelling, real feminism isn't about male hatred or replacing men. Simply put, feminism is an ideology and movement whose primary goal is to dismantle a system of hierarchical oppression based on gender superiority, colloquially referred to as "patriarchy." Don't let the word throw you off. Any studied feminist will be the first to tell you that this system isn't good for men either, and feminism is, in fact, fighting for the well-being of men as well as women. Furthermore, feminism doesn't suggest that just because you're a man you're a terrible human being.

Unfortunately, some feminist schools of thought in the 1960s and 1970s did have tones of anti-male sentiment and sadly, among some communities, feminism as a whole has never recovered. As a result, contemporary intersectional feminism, no matter how spot-on, has a marketing problem. It gets twisted by those who argue in bad faith to perpetuate the myth that feminism is inherently anti-male. The information is being too easily dismissed and rejected because just the words *feminism* and *patriarchy* have become so loaded and misunderstood.

My calves are muddy and cramped after another long day of training. I'm sitting on the edge of my bed in front of a mess of enlarged images of Everest that I use to keep me motivated. I used to be able to stare at them for hours trying to memorize every rock and vein of ice. These days, however, I'm too distracted, still trying to unwind what happened and the storm of emotion inside me. Instead of studying the pictures, I catch myself staring vacantly at an aloe plant. The fleshy leaves are plump and soft, protected by sharp, serrated edges. The furnace hums and Rupert is licking my ear and I think that this isn't just about me and my brain. There is something universal in this mess. We all make mistakes. We all misstep. We all offend. Every gender. But in the context of sexuality, it's mostly men and I wonder why.

The majority of abuse resulting from patriarchal culture *is* perpetrated by men against women. In other ways, patriarchy harms men in astonishing numbers as well. It starts young as we're taught that boys are strong. Boys don't cry. Boys don't express except through competition and channeled aggression. Good boys become strong leaders by repressing emotion under a façade of false stoicism. By initiating boys into antiquated gender roles, we're asked to divorce ourselves from our fullest emotional expression because that kind of vulnerability isn't "strong" or "safe." In doing so, our emotional development is stunted and our long-term capacity for connection and intimacy along with it. In time, boys become men who have bottled up a lifetime of pain until eventually we boil over. In this system, anger becomes the primary male emotion, which pushes away the very connection we long for. When anger abounds, love is eroded by fear.

Because Mom was the breadwinner, I always thought that I'd somehow inherited feminism. It's just another way I misunderstood. Equal access to wealth and power is only a fraction of what feminism is fighting for. If it stops there, all we've done is replace who's making the money, which doesn't address the deeper underlying issues.

Still, men hold most of the wealth and the power it affords. Because of this, money and status are reinforced as the highest calling of masculine desirability. While this has some biological underpinnings, to men, providing women with "safety" has become a misunderstood reason for being. It's a false path to love.

When that path inevitably leaves us emotionally isolated (rich and powerful, poor and "weak," or somewhere in between), men often turn toward the other realm of conditioned masculinity: we try to extract power and/or emotional connection through sexuality.

Isolation and anger are two primary drivers for unchecked, aggressive sexual behavior, from pornography abuse to prostitution, coercion, and rape—and, yes, even something as seemingly "benign" as a nonconsensual slap on the ass. Now, I'm being forced to ask if my actions were expressions of power that I always had but never understood. At their deepest roots? Yes. And there is nothing benign about it.

What finally makes me understand aren't the books and articles I'm reading. I only really get it when I start asking the women in my life about their experiences. I used to ask as a way to offer a rebuttal and to assert myself and my opinion. Now I'm asking without waiting for my turn to respond. When I start listening and let go of my "what-about-isms," I finally get it.

Once I finally start to see it, like so many men in the wake of the #MeToo movement, I'm forced into contemplation regarding my own actions, recalling and turning over and chewing on my entire history. What might I have done to make someone feel uncomfortable? What presumptions might I have made and how might my actions have been interpreted in ways that I never intended or imagined? How, and how many times, have I misunderstood?

Patriarchy is not a problem that gets solved in a decade. Gender roles and identities are our inheritance as much as any material possessions. They're just much harder to get rid of. In a moment of radical cultural upheaval, rapidly shifting definitions cause jarring social disruptions and I see that I'm not the only one who has misunderstood or is confused. Daphne Merkin continues, "We need a broader and more thorough-going overhaul, one that begins with the way we bring up our sons and daughters." It takes time.

As it exists today, patriarchy is not a system strictly upheld or enabled by men. It's entrenched in our entire culture and learned by all genders from a very young age. We learn it from books and movies and mothers and fathers alike. This doesn't excuse the abuse of women at the hands of men. Many of us are simply blind to how we contribute and perpetuate it. If that's hard to swallow for some, we need look no further than the beauty industry that dominates our culture and the overwhelming pressure women face to look a certain way. By literally buying into a patriarchal view of what they "should" look like to be desirable to get the rich and powerful partner for social and economic status and "safety," the cycle continues. There's a natural, biological element to this, and there is nothing wrong with beauty as an expression of any gender. We need to attract partners. Ideas of beauty are dynamic and change over time. The issue is how those ideas are manipulated and used to reinforce sexist gender roles. This is just one example.

Feminist pioneer and thinker bell hooks was bold and ruffled a lot of feathers in *The Will to Change* when she wrote:

> We need to highlight the role women play in perpetuating and sustaining patriarchal culture so that we will recognize patriarchy as a system women and men support equally, even if men receive more rewards from that system. Dismantling and changing patriarchal culture is work that men and women must do together.

The rewards she speaks of are muddy at times as is evidenced by the rate of male suicide (more coming on that). For me, I'm beginning to see that those rewards are often best understood by what I as a man *don't* experience versus what I do. She was also

abundantly clear that this in no way excuses the abuse perpetrated by men:

> It does not erase or lessen male responsibility for supporting
> and perpetuating their power under patriarchy to exploit and
> oppress women in a manner far more grievous than the seri-
> ous psychological stress and emotional pain caused by male
> conformity to rigid sexist role patterns.

As is made so clear by hooks, we all suffer from patriarchy and
the onus of change rests in *all* of our hands. And yet the majority
of the work is still being done by women. It's a cruel irony that
the oppressed are somehow responsible for breaking their own
chains.

The goal is not to raise one sex and/or gender above or at the
cost of another but to dismantle the systems of oppression that
harm us all. Matriarchy is just another system of gender superiority no matter how tempting it might be to suggest it's a better
system. Drawing parallels to our primate cousins or the enclaves
where it exists is a reductive, albeit seductive, argument. It's also
worth pointing out that as much as the system we live in has
traded on and led to oppression, it has also made its positive
contributions. Like so much, it's not all good and it's not all bad,
and it's important not to throw the baby out with the bathwater.

Regarding mental health, however, as I begin to understand
the abuses enabled by the underbelly of patriarchy, I see a bottomless ocean of trauma. Eventually power imbalances result in
conflict and violence. Violence begets trauma and trauma is the
root of mental health issues. Any system of gender (or racial, religious, political, etc.) superiority will always lead to conflict.

Because we live in a patriarchal culture, it's reasonable then to
point to imbalances of oppression as the source of the vast majority of cultural sickness, from climate change and war to abuse

and violence in the home and on the street. Put bluntly, unchecked patriarchy (and other systemic inequalities, if they can even be separated) is likely the greatest cause of the mental health crisis today.

If we are to begin to really address mental health as a collective, these systemic inequalities must die.

Obviously, not all sexual humor needs to be litigated, and not every spank is sexual. We shouldn't be afraid to hug each other. We shouldn't be afraid to flirt. It's also okay to admit we're wrong and we shouldn't be afraid of the nuances when we miss the mark. A society of eggshells ends up in pieces, and a black-and-white world makes no room for understanding. It makes no space for the messiness of being human. It leaves no room for forgiveness or discourse or healing or progress.

Dismantling these systems of oppression is an uphill battle made more difficult because just the words *patriarchy* and *feminism* have become so polarized that many people simply shut off when they hear them. I did. It's not the stories of feminism and patriarchy that need to change, but it's worth considering the language we're using to tell them.

We can't just shrug this off as "male fragility" either (if for no other reason than the whole idea of male fragility echoes patriarchy's foundational rejection of male emotion). None of this should be political and there is no "wokeness" here. The "crisis of masculinity" is itself reflective of reimagining how we can navigate the world together with more equity. There is no left and right, as the angry man on the internet wants us to believe. The words themselves have been politicized by *all* sides.

Working for *National Geographic* was a massive piece of my identity and life. It feels close enough to touch, but it's already out of reach and drifting farther away. The remaining pieces of my identity feel fragile, and I wonder if there is any way to climb out of this. I study pictures of Everest and feel hope and fear and put on my running tights and Rupert sniffs me all over and cocks his head a bit to the left.

It's been seven years since the incident and a year and a half since the lawyer called. A pandemic is raging, a Black man named George Floyd has been murdered in the street, and the world of storytelling has been rightfully upended to make room for new, more diverse voices. That's good. Regardless, I feel a massive void and I'm unsure what can fill it up. I put on my running shoes.

I call Dad from the car on my way to the trailhead and ask him if he's dead yet. "Ohhhhh, not yet." I ask if he's enjoying his grim reaper T-shirt. He tells me he's wearing it at the hardware store because he needs to fix a door and I think he must be very happy buying screws. I ask if it's an entrance or an exit and he laughs because he loves words as much as me and says, "Yes." I tell him that the case is closed.

"Do you think you'll ever work for them again?"

"I don't know. I hope so."

"This too shall pass."

"I love you."

"Go gently." He hangs up in a tangle of loud sounds the way old people do and goes home to fix the exit that is also an entrance.

32

I have a paper cut from writing my suicide note.

It's a start. . . .

—STEVEN WRIGHT

It's dawn and the world is pink and quiet. Tiny snow crystals are floating upward, weightlessly crossing through the shadows of trees and shafts of light. It's –10°F and the snow is loud under my boots. I was here yesterday, and the day before, and the day before that, following the same trail to the same mountains, always alone. But I don't mind. I'm alone most days now. Rupert isn't allowed in Rocky Mountain National Park, and besides, he's not much of a climber.

After an hour I cross a broad meadow of short, twisted trees that look like a sculpture gallery. Behind me the thrust of the Rockies falls away in faded layers, flattening into the eastward plains. I think of what the world looked like before us. I picture the first people wandering across the landscape, seeing this for the first time and how quiet it must have been. Quiet like now.

The dirt is frozen and hard, blown over by thin snow. My boots crunch on the exposed gravel as the orange granite of Longs Peak glows above the blue ice of Chasm Lake. I hop from boulder to boulder and my climbing boots feel awkward and clunky. After another hour I put on my crampons and pull on my harness and take my ice axes from the pack and begin connecting the tiny edges of stone that I've memorized. The climbing isn't hard, but the climbing on Everest won't be either and I spin lyrics in my head like I always do. After forty minutes the lake is 2,000 feet below me, in shade. I swing my ice axes into thin ice that I know will hold my weight but my heart quickens all the same as I scrape and pull and think it would be an awfully long fall. It doesn't really matter how hard the terrain is when you're climbing without a rope. One mistake is always too many. I hear only myself and the voice in my head and the wind.

When I get to the ridge, my phone comes alive with messages and missed calls. But I see only one. Topo says, "Everest season is canceled again." I sit and close my eyes and wipe sweat from my forehead and run my fingers through greasy hair. It's 2021 and we've been training relentlessly for two years to go back. Last year the season was canceled by the pandemic. With nothing else to do, it made sense to just keep working toward the goal. Today the news strikes me differently and I feel a bit hollow, wondering how much more I have and how much longer I can survive on the money left in the bank. I pick at frozen chocolate on my jacket and text Topo: "What do we do now?"

He texts back: "I have an idea."

A month later, Tommy Joyce and I land in Kathmandu. To me, the smells and colors are familiar. An unending tangle of scooters and cars flows through a scattershot of cows, dogs, people, dust, and shrines. Women in bright sarees balance baskets on their heads and dart across the road while dirt-covered kids scamper after them or panhandle outside the windows of cars. Buddhists thumb prayer beads and their lips move silently, repeating mantras over and over again, and I wonder if they ever get bored. The air is thick with sweat and incense and smoke from Hindus burning their dead. Even on the clearest days and despite all the color, I always picture the city under a lazy, yellow mist. The roads are more knotted than organized and even after nearly twenty trips here I still get lost and it all feels like a strange, sweaty hug. I try to count every trip and watch Tommy while the driver swerves around holy cows, draped in necklaces of flowers, that like to eat garbage in the middle of the road. For Tommy, everything is new and I wish I could see it all for the first time again.

Tommy is 5'10", 165 pounds, and as big as a house. He's farmboy strong and has a broad jaw under blue eyes and sandy brows and moves decisively. He's playful, gifted, and fiercely sharp, as if life hasn't been able to catch up and dull his edges or quiet his voice. He seems certain of everything. Above all, he's talented and relentless.

For the past eight months Keith Ladzinski, Tommy, and I have been working on the film about my life. It's a film about cancer and loss and the messiness of family and the mind, all set against the audacious goal of trying to climb a new route on the highest mountain in the world. It's a compelling pitch and the project has consumed everyone involved.

We've spent hundreds of hours filming, learning about narrative structure, and dissecting the story of family and life, and it's bonded us . . . especially Tommy and me. He's with me when I train. When I take my pills and go to bed. When I go to the doctor and have blood drawn. He's up early and in bed late every day, diligently documenting every moment of my life. But it's not just me. By now Tommy knows my family as well as anyone.

My mouth tastes like a twenty-four-hour flight when we arrive at the hotel and crawl from the minibus. Topo and his girlfriend, Carla, are standing in a heap of duffels and blue plastic barrels and I can smell the musk of climbing gear and rope that's been in storage for two years. We hug and I hold his face.

"Que tal?" It's all the Spanish I know.

"Todo bien." He smiles, and we hug again.

The next days are filled up with permits and diplomatic meetings. Our permit to climb a new route on Dhaulagiri, the seventh-highest mountain in the world, is granted. It will be a dry run for Everest in 2022.

The days in Kathmandu are hot and humid, strung together by hours of conversation and packing. Tommy films as Topo and Carla and I sit in our rooms and sort through thousands of pounds of colorful gear and food we'll need for six weeks on the mountain. I've done this a thousand times and it happens mechanically, leaving me to my thoughts, which seem a little fast. I fall asleep at 6 P.M. and wake up at 11 and watch Bollywood films on TV and never go back to sleep. After a week I'm sleeping less and less. I'm easily teary and forcing myself to eat. But none of this seems out of place. I'm just tired from the travel. I'm just jet-lagged. I am just fine.

The helicopter whines and we're weightless as the jungle falls away into smoke from thick forest fires that are ravaging the foothills. We angle left into a steep gorge and I see lone figures winding their way up trails that cut across hillsides and I'm very happy we aren't walking. Eventually the trees give way to barren steppes and the river becomes braided strips of white ice that weave and wind and come back together in statuesque waterfalls. The helicopter dips into the shade and the mountain swallows the view. Of all the 8,000-meter peaks I've seen, Dhaulagiri appears as the biggest and fiercest—and much, much harder than Everest.

The engine shifts and the world slows. I jump from the door into the rotor wash as crystals of snow are blasted against my face and melt. My thoughts are very fast.

The first night we sleep in the cook tent and I listen to everyone shift and snore. Their breathing is sporadic, swelling with big, deep breaths until it stops altogether and I wait for the anxious inhale that will eventually follow. This kind of labored breathing is called Cheyne-Stokes respiration and can be terrifying for people who've never felt its rhythm. I know it's a normal adaptation to the altitude and it reminds me where I am and it all feels normal. What I don't understand is why I can't sleep at all.

We spend two days digging and moving boulders to level out small platforms for our tents. The northwest ridge above us looms heavy in black and white. It towers and seems violent. Avalanches and rockfall dislodge and crash and thunder because, like Everest, the earth here is new and unsettled.

After three days my edges feel dull and hard, like all the soft pieces of my body have worn off. There's a pervasive sense of weightlessness and vertigo. I sleep less and less until I'm sick in my tent, unable to breathe through my nose. The COVID tests are negative but I isolate myself anyway and tell the team I'm fine. I just need to heal for a day. Just need to rest. I tell them I'm okay. I am anything but.

Tonight I don't sleep. Have I ever slept? I stare at the nylon ceiling and count the tiny squares. I close my eyes and try to meditate as the world spins in the old familiar flashes of black and white, formless and sharp and chaotic. There are no words and too many letters and memories and thoughts that don't connect. I try to read but the sentences don't end. When I piece together a page, I start to cry for no reason and the tears pool in my ears. I pray and apologize and clutch and claw, yet everything seems to be circling a black hole. I write pages of bad stand-up comedy and think I'm very funny and imagine myself standing onstage. I'll have a Netflix special and flirt with Ali Wong. As quickly as one daydream fades another begins, and now I'm on the mountain, just as excited about dying as about standing on top. Now I'm a movie star. And now I am yelling at trees in a park. Fantasy and nightmares and noise and it's terribly quiet everywhere but behind my eyes.

In the morning I'm much sicker. My sinuses are packed with thick yellow mucus and I'm sweating. The team goes to explore the access to the lower face while I lie in my sleeping bag and blow my nose until it bleeds. I listen to the wind brush through camp, interrupted by the occasional avalanche or rockslide. Aside from that, everything is blanketed in an uneasy silence. I hug my legs to my chest and bounce my jaw on my knees, rocking back and forth and holding my head. I can't stop crying but am startled to notice that I'm crying at all. At some point I start talking to myself in measured tones, assuring myself that everything is okay. But eventually the only words that are coming out are "I'm sorry" and "No, no, no." I start screaming as loud as I can into my sleeping bag, trying to muffle what's unfolding inside me, clutching my chest as my heart beats and I'm too alive . . . too keenly aware of everything. I know, feel, and understand that no piece of this life works for me anymore. I'm not a climber. I'm not a photographer. But if I'm not these things, it means I'm formless.

Now I'm repeating "I love you" over and over and over and have no idea whom I'm talking to. I love everything, as if the universe is running through me. My mind swims in overwhelming currents of emotion that I can neither define nor ignore. I love the big down jacket that keeps me almost comfortable. I love the smell of melted snow in my tin cup. I love the pile of Nepali off-brand condiments on the dining tent table. Peanut Butter & Co. Since 1998. Druk Tomato Ketchup and the mountain moans. I love them all so much. None of this tracks. It's so beautiful it literally hurts and I'm very confused because all I can think of is dying. Now I'm laughing. Now I'm crying. Now I'm screaming and now I'm quiet, staring at bubbles of water on my mattress. It takes minutes before I understand that they are my own tears.

Right now I'm fixated on the idea that this is all about an identity that I'm shedding. All I see is that the life I've been living no longer works. And it's true. It doesn't. I've been trying to shove myself into a box that I no longer fit. It's a beautiful life of adventure and art and bigger and bigger mountains. It's all I know and I can't imagine what is beyond its confines because what will I be if I am not this? Will I exist at all?

I text a friend and tell her, "I feel like I am swimming against every fiber of my being. I see the beauty but I can't feel anything. . . . My identity and ego are clashing against a reality that this life doesn't serve me anymore. . . . I'm so scared of what it means to let this go." As if she can sense the severity of the situation and my fear, she responds simply: "The biggest risk is to let it go, be honest, and find out that you are still loved."

I send more messages, casting a net for a lifeline, but no one responds right away because it's midnight back home. Eventually I get a text back from Laurel, my therapist, encouraging me to leave the mountains. To her, something about my words and situation seems off. Finally I text my brother and say the same thing: "I can't. I'm done. None of this works. I'm so scared. I'm fucked." We hardly communicate at all these days, so I'm surprised when my phone buzzes with a response: "You'll make the right decision. Stay strong. I love you." Three words I've waited for my whole life. I wonder how many times he's wanted to say them but held back, saving them for this moment. A lifeboat. A rope. Hold on.

When the team returns, we sit in the dining tent and I tell them I'm done. I give them no warning and, as is expected with unexpected news, I'm answered with shock. It's as confusing as it is absurd and they stare at me as if I've lost my mind. It's not as simple as leaving an expedition. I'm telling them that I have to change everything . . . that this life is over. I don't want to climb. I don't want to take pictures. I want to move to California and start over and it all seems insane.

Topo breathes heavily while I hold my breath. The others in the tent stare at their feet, at us, at nothing at all, avoiding the crossfire of disdain, love, and feeble excuses. But it's unavoidable. I understand his anger. Poised beneath the seventh-highest mountain in the world attempting a climb that has never been done before, a film crew in place, and a hundred thousand dollars spent, pulling out now is unhinged. I'm also stamping out our shared dream of Everest and torching brotherhood, the very bond I hold most dear.

My brain spins in a thousand directions, egged on by a hypomanic state that I can neither identify nor understand. There are two very real things happening simultaneously but somehow I only see one of them. It's true that I need to close this chapter of my life. It's true that the stress of this world of motion and risk has run its course and that I can no longer choose to live in madness to escape it. This I know. What I can't see is that finally, in this moment, the madness has caught up and overtaken me.

My confession lasts thirty minutes until no one has anything left to say. I leave the team in shock and walk through darkness to my tent. The soft voices behind me aren't clear but I know what they are saying. I don't care. After twenty years all I want is to rest. I crawl into my sleeping bag and close my eyes and stare.

My body is lifeless but my eyes are very blue and bloodshot. They bulge from a purple face. Dormant veins hold dark, pooled blood. I'm naked, suspended from a piece of climbing rope hanging from the ceiling. The cord that has tethered me to life is finally choking me out. The birds sing outside the windows. A tiny layer of dust has formed over every surface. No one will find me for days and finally my brain is quiet. I am at peace.

I don't sleep again, wishing minutes into hours until finally the sun comes up. We say very little to each other. Topo hugs me and says, "I love you. I just want the best for you," and I apologize to everyone. Tommy is kind and Carla is sweet and I walk away and follow the braided river down the valley alone.

———————

Back in Colorado a week later, I watch a colorless orchid hover over my head, nodding in the current of air from the heater. The shapes of the apartment blend in dark chunks. It's too early for Mom to be calling but I still haven't slept, so I answer and she asks, "Have you seen the email?" I put her on speaker and open a scathing message from Tommy, accusing me of a vast, calculated manipulation. It's to my parents and me and everyone involved in the film. All she can say is, "Cory, I don't understand." But I do. He's furious and hurt and I understand the anger. He and Keith and Topo and our producer, Emma, have dedicated countless hours and effort and opened themselves completely. They feel betrayed. Mom feels the same. She's opened her home and given her time and dredged through painful memories for the film, all at my request. Somehow I still can't see what's happening and there's no recognition that this might be related to my mind. But I have disrupted life so completely for so many people that I see only one clear solution.

I shower for somewhere between two minutes and an hour because I want to be clean when they find me.

I grab a green climbing rope from the mudroom.

I Google "how to tie a noose" and stand naked and practice and I like the shape.

I admire the symmetry and think it's a very handsome knot and Dad would be proud.

I notice my hands that look like Mom's.

I think I need a stool.

I climb on top and am quite relieved that this will all be over soon.

I notice my bent second toes and think of my brother and how he will inherit all my things.

I put the rope around my neck and gently lean onto the noose.

My carotid artery pulses in my neck and my eyes begin to bulge. My fantasy is coming to life.

I lean harder until I can't breathe and hang until I feel my eyes begin to blink closed.

. . .

Just before I black out, I reach for the rope above my head and pull.

The stool wobbles.

The stool tips.

. . .

I catch it between my feet and hold on.

. . .

I crawl off the stool and sit.

I shake.

I look at the orchid above my bed.

I don't want to die. I just don't want to live like this.

. . .

I send an SOS to space and back. Help.

I hear a knock on the door.

My friend Lori drapes over my lower back and her blond hair falls off my waist and she says, "Don't go." I feel her own tears sandwiched between her cheek and my skin. Her head feels like a heavy, warm stone anchoring me to the world. I feel her hand in my hair. She guards me from my ghosts and I drift away and finally sleep deep and hard.

Here are some not-so-fun facts from the CDC: In 2020, 45,979 people killed themselves in the United States. That's one death every eleven minutes. From 2000 to 2018, suicides increased 36 percent. Nearly 80 percent of all those deaths were men. Worldwide, men account for about 71 percent of suicides. This suggests not that men are weaker but rather that we feel our suf-

fering is best kept hidden. In hiding, we become the casualties of
the system we built.

For me, suicidal ideation has always been tied to my depressive swings. My current dance with it is clearly tied to the fallout
of my rapid exit from an entire life and career and the bipolar
episode that precipitated it. But it's obvious that something else
is going on. The rising rate of suicide and mental health issues in
the country as a whole is likely tied to a pandemic, and not just
the one floating through the empty streets forcing unnatural isolation and an addiction to our screens. We live in a world of toxic
stress.

Both social media and the twenty-four-hour news cycle saturate us with a near-constant bombardment of seemingly hopeless and often false information, increasing toxic stress, which is
linked to mental health issues, which is linked to suicide, and if
you don't see that connection, your eyes are closed.

Excessive social media use is directly tied to increased rates of
depression. One study by the University of Utah found that teens
who use social media are as much as three times as likely to suffer
from depression, amplifying the risk of attempted suicide and
death. According to the CDC, suicide is now the second-leading
cause of death for individuals ten to thirty-four years old. Another study by researchers at Brigham Young University pointed
out that the use of social media in teens disproportionately affects girls and I wonder again about what flawed masculinity
teaches young women about their value.

For my own part, I think about #EverestNoFilter and think
#HairByEverest might be the same look as #HairByDepression.
I wonder if my voice has contributed to a flawed narrative of
perfection in a culture of comparison. Has it been inspirational
or damaging? Both? I've also used social media to build my platform to talk about mental health. Have I helped anyone?

Thumb through social media enough, though, and eventually

you'll read this: "Hard times create strong men. Strong men create good times. Good times create weak men. And weak men create hard times." The quote is from *Those Who Remain* by G. Michael Hopf. The implication is that times are easy now and everyone is too soft, which is creating hard times. And if times are so easy, maybe the role of everyone is to just shut up. Be stronger. After all, your grandfather went to war and never said a thing, right?

It's true the "developed" world is no longer walking uphill both ways to factory jobs and making pennies. A hundred and fifty years ago they used a bone saw with no anesthetic to remove limbs. There was the Dust Bowl and the Great Depression and two world wars. Times were hard and sacrifices were made. But to suggest that our younger generations are soft because the older generations were so tough is flawed. Since I was born, the United States has been at war at least three times, the Twin Towers fell, the economy collapsed. A pandemic swept, acts of domestic terrorism are climbing, climate change rages, and it seems like every week someone walks into a school and starts shooting. If you think we are a weak society creating hard times, you're one generation behind. We live in a world of constant stress and it's being yelled at us through every screen at every hour of the day.

Saying times are hard now does not dismiss the struggles of the past. It's important to ask if, perhaps, all generations have their unique battles and advantages. It's also human nature for older generations to regale younger ones with their sacrifice and point to how easy the next generation has it. It's a nostalgic trope as old as humans. But there's a serious problem with it.

When we tell people they "have it easy" in the moment when they take the risk of expressing themselves, it flatly denies their emotional experience, driving disconnection and eroding safety to express ourselves in the future. A sense of perspective is important, but the depth of our suffering is relative not to what others have endured but to our own experiences. We know others have it harder, but neurobiologically our suffering is equal. The way to lend perspective is to validate the emotional experience first. Once it's acknowledged, the brain can move out of the stress response and reengage reason and logic. It still doesn't allow us to know the subjective experience of another's suffering, but it can give a frame of reference for our own. Only once we're there can we shift toward gratitude for what we do have instead of focusing on what we don't.

Speaking about pain, anger, frustration, and everything else isn't weak and it doesn't make anyone a "snowflake." It requires real vulnerability, which is a skill of strength. When emotions are shared, it shows deep trust. It can feel burdensome to help carry the load of another's pain, but it's also an honor to be trusted and asked. Engaging with the suffering of others, especially when it challenges our own experiences and stories, takes courage. Empathy requires vulnerability and it's one of the strongest things in the world. It connects us, and together we can all endure more. In silence, we collapse. In silence, we die.

33

"Asking for help isn't giving up," said the horse.

"It's refusing to give up."

—CHARLIE MACKESY, *The Boy, the Mole, the Fox and the Horse*

The psychiatrist sits at a big wooden desk covered in papers and the room is bright. He's kind but not overly sensitive as he scribbles notes and I wonder what they say. Finally he looks at me gravely and says, "Cory, you've had a very, very serious mixed bipolar episode. All the revelations about your path and life may be very honest, but your neurobiology is also playing a profound role in your perception. If you don't get a handle on this *now*, it will likely get worse over time." I wonder how much of my life has been shaped by undiagnosed episodes as he continues, "Do you know what triggered it?"

"Well, my dad has terminal cancer. I've recently lost a big piece of my job, which I guess is also sort of my identity. But it's also pretty financially stressful. Ummm, I've been making a film. I've been training fifteen to twenty hours a week for a year for a new route on Everest and I think a lot about dying. Shit, I mean the pandemic. I flew across the world and my sleep cycle got all fucked up and I never really recovered. I'm a little heartsick from a recent breakup and I've been—"

"Stop," he interrupts. He means two things.

Two days later, a nurse attaches sticky patches to my chest and I think they're going to rip out a lot of chest hair. She wraps the blood pressure cuff around my arm and it inflates and clicks and throbs with my heartbeat as she writes down the numbers in a little pad and asks, "Are you warm? Do you have an eye mask? Are you comfortable?" I have almost no energy to speak and nod as I watch a needle slip into my vein.

The nurse attaches a bag of clear fluid to the IV and says, "Just relax," which is never a good sign. She turns a plastic clip and I watch the ketamine fill a long tube and slip its way into my veins and I blast off to another planet, like I'm at the best music festival and all my favorite bands are playing at once. It's dark behind the eye mask and I can't tell if I'm asleep or awake or dreaming. I don't know if all the dark fractals in front of my open eyes are real or make-believe and I wonder where the earth has gone. My right and left hands feel confused, disconnected from my arms, which have disappeared altogether.

Psychedelics and plant medicine have been around for eons from the Amazon to ancient Greece and Egypt and nearly everywhere else. In history they were a vehicle for transcendence that opened doors to a broader perception of the nature of reality and its intersection with the divine. Some have gone so far as to suggest that it was psychedelic experiences that planted the philosophical seeds for thinkers like Plato, Cicero, and Marcus Aurelius. It's even been suggested, with considerable evidence, that Christianity itself is tied to a psychedelic carryover from Eleusis, the "spiritual capital of the ancient world."

Psychedelic experience and research exploded again in the 1950s and 1960s and found its way into pop culture, only to be quickly demonized. Through criminalization, the reputation of psychedelics was severely damaged, with them characterized as "drugs that will make you crazy." It took another thirty to forty years for their uses to be broadly reexamined, especially as they relate to mental health. But it was always suspected that there was more to the story. Bill Wilson, the co-founder of Alcoholics Anonymous, was a strong believer in the power of LSD to free the deeply addicted and the ongoing research is promising to say the least. Just read Michael Pollan's *How to Change Your Mind*.

Unlike traditional pharmaceuticals, which focus on the symptoms of mental health issues, psychedelics seem to restructure, reignite, and positively alter the neural pathways that have been damaged. Rather than dumping a whole bunch of oil on the engine to grease the pistons of the brain, psychedelics appear to help restructure the engine block altogether.

They do seem to have *real* impacts on depression and anxiety. Ketamine in particular has been shown to be a wildly successful interventional therapy for treatment-resistant depression. But psychedelics aren't for everyone, especially those who have a history with psychosis. Bipolar is stickier because of the fear of resultant mania, but the research is promising and gaining speed.

It's a very unregulated world and there is *a lot* of misinformation as well as pseudo–spiritual healers who have no understanding of the mechanisms of the brain and neurobiology. Uneducated practitioners and facilitators run the real risk of creating more trauma and not everyone on Instagram is trustworthy.

At their best, psychedelics seem to lift people from years of sadness, pain, addiction, and trauma. At their worst, they conflate experience with healing, enable spiritual and emotional bypassing, and can *cause* deep trauma without informed guidance. The "wounded healer" is a real thing and altered states are ripe fields for abuse. With so many people "facilitating" psychedelics and heralding their healing properties, it's easy to imagine them as a panacea. A hack to healing. They aren't.

Psychedelics are not a cure and just because we have an amazing experience and begin to understand ourselves more wholly, it does not mean that we are healed. I know lots of people who have done ayahuasca thirty times and are still flaming assholes, incapable of sitting with their own pain or that of others.

Understanding the origins of our trauma is only the first step and if we're not careful we can get stuck there. Understanding helps us form a rough structure around ourselves and our journey with pathologies, behaviors, thought patterns, and mental health. But the story itself isn't healing. Healing comes when we transcend the story altogether and divorce ourselves from its negative influences. Integration means dropping the story because the story no longer informs your actions.

Doing peyote in the desert might be fun and enlightening. There's nothing wrong with it. But it likely isn't having the impact you think regarding mental health. Don't mistake a dream about making fire for knowing how to do it when you're awake. You've got the information; now go rub some sticks together. Do it over and over and over. Psychedelic therapist Lauren Taus reminds us that, "Life isn't a cognitive exercise. It's an action sport. Understanding isn't enough. You have to go out and do the damn thing."

Most often, deep healing and lasting therapeutic benefits rely on set, setting, and guidance. It takes time and it's good to be wary of anyone telling you different. Lasting change simply does not happen overnight. Psychedelics can set us on the path, but it's our responsibility to walk it. If you change nothing, nothing will change long-term, no matter how many times you go to space.

After an hour in orbit, the ground rushes toward me and I feel the chair underneath me, gently catching the fall. My cheeks are wet and my mouth is dry. Reality feels like a warm blanket. The nurse gives me some apple juice and I tip up awkwardly to drink and think I really need to pee. She peels back the sticky pads and it feels like fire ants and I'm a little angry because I like my chest hair. "How do you feel?"

I do six ketamine infusions over two weeks and I'm lifted. The suicidal thoughts fade and finally disappear. My mind is slow and measured and the sharp edges of the world are gone. It's not too much to say that ketamine saves my life. It's like a hard reboot. I'm smiling and joking and it seems to happen overnight. Everyone is saying, "You seem . . . different." I'm no longer swimming with ankle weights on. I'm not in the sea at all. For the first time I can remember, I'm on the beach enjoying the view. I feel gratitude for life, as if I'm remembering something I didn't know I forgot. The only word I can find for the experience is *normal,* and normal has never felt so special. I wake up somehow new. The orchid is bouncing overhead and I see that it's pink.

Keith Ladzinski, my co-director on the Everest film, is tall and dark with smart-looking glasses and straight hair that combs itself. I have known him for almost twenty years. He talks with his hands and listens to audiobooks like I listen to music and his brain is filled with big ideas. His photography and film are exacting, as if he's trying to wring out every drop of natural beauty in the world. I've always envied his relentless creativity. His humor is dry and quick and he can twist anything into a joke. We've only had one disagreement in our friendship, when I couldn't find my gloves and thought he might have misplaced them (I was sitting on them). He's opened a thousand doors for me.

We've been in business together and have traveled all over the world making art and I remember teaching him how to ski in Antarctica. We spent forty-six days alone on the ice while he chased snow petrels with his camera. I think of how I told him about the history of Tibet as we drove across the Tibetan Plateau en route to Everest in 2019. It all feels a million miles away while we walk under a canopy of cottonwood trees with coffee.

"I'm sorry," I say.

"I know. This wasn't okay, man. We've put in hundreds of hours and lots of dollars on this film." He pauses as we step over cracks in the concrete, pushed up by roots and grass. But he's thoughtful with his words because he's been witness to the wreckage of mental illness in his own life, and he continues, "I know it isn't your 'fault' that you're a psychotic mess." I love his humor even more and we laugh. "I know it's more complex than that. I love you all the same." I think I'm lucky to have friends like him. I know too that he'll likely never trust me again and I understand because mental health issues are exhausting.

A few weeks later, *The New York Times* publishes "Should a Mental Health Emergency Derail a Dangerous Climb?" by Kelley Manley. Whether or not mental health "should" or "shouldn't" derail anything misses the point, but the article is fair and balanced and reads like a tennis match.

Tommy, Topo, and Carla release a joint statement that says, "The sport is too dangerous to have mental insecurity, especially at altitude." I wonder what that means for every successful expedition I've been on. By that logic, I should have never pursued climbing and alpinism should be reserved for the "strong of mind." It implies a fundamental weakness and reinforces the flawed story of masculinity. By that logic, no one who has ever suffered from depression or anxiety or bipolar should go on big adventures, even if it's healthy for them. My answer to this volleys back, "What people with these struggles need is more participation, more engagement in order to understand that mental health issues aren't prohibitive of living a full and complete life."

The article continues with Tommy saying, "I think he figured that he could leave and go back to being a 'mental health advocate.' Cory had to create a new narrative that protected his ego from his ever-present fear that he doesn't matter." Topo says, "Plenty of athletes have mental health issues that don't affect their performance. The lack of accountability and commitment is what bothers me the most." Both statements sting.

Tommy is making an astute observation that I have a deep need to "matter." Much of my life and career has been about exactly that, but it hurts to see it in black and white, no matter how many times I've said it. However, I've been publicly discussing mental health since 2016 and this is not a new narrative.

But the idea that I am using mental health to escape accountability, as Topo is hinting, is troubling. I swing back: "If I'd broken my leg, the conversation would be, 'Well, that's a bummer, sometimes you go into the mountains and things happen.' But because mental health is a topic of the mind and is unseen except through behavior, it's nearly incomprehensible for people to apply the same logic and objectivity to it. I can't demand that the world understands my experience, but I can ask that they believe it's true."

It's as if all my transparency and advocacy around mental health has been one long scream into a void. In a moment of crisis, even my closest friends can't grasp that everything I've spoken of is real despite the blatant display I've just offered. But how can I really expect them to understand? It occurs to me that true understanding can only come through embodiment and I really don't wish that on anyone. It's my responsibility to understand them even though I know they can never fully understand me.

With persistent mental health issues like bipolar, the capacity of friends and loved ones to weather the ups and downs can diminish over time. Those ups and downs can't be seen like a broken leg or scoliosis or cancer; instead, they are often seen as a choice.

The idea that the behaviors surrounding mental health issues are as simple as choice is both true and false. Like everything, the truth is somewhere in the middle. Someone enraptured in a bipolar episode *might* be able to see their actions, but just as likely they can't. Even if they do, behaviors that seem baffling to someone else are reflexive and probably totally "logical" to the person making the decisions. It's only when the episode has abated that the oddity of everything is revealed. Again, and I can't stress this enough, it doesn't excuse anything because the choices are still our own. In fact, accountability and a thorough accounting of everything are necessary to change the patterns. The problem is that the consequences of the actions can be so painful and destructive that people fall away before the patterns can change and I hear another friend say, "I just can't deal with you any longer." All I can say is, "Okay," and stop calling them when it's dark. I call someone else and they say, "Can I call you back?" I wait for the phone to ring. When it doesn't, I take the point.

Even more frustrating is that often the shift to stability happens quickly. I was nearly suicidal yesterday, but today everything is normal. Yesterday I wouldn't shut up, but today I am calm. That the severity of a situation can change so quickly reinforces the idea that someone is making informed, deliberate choices and looks a bit like someone crying wolf. I think it's no wonder everyone around me is tired and confused and stops answering. I would. I have.

Some people do try to escape accountability by hiding behind the shield of an unstable mind. It's an easy excuse and manipulation. I've done it. But this is not that and there is no piece of me that's trying to escape the responsibility of Dhaulagiri. It's easy to understand why they would think that I was hiding behind it because my understanding came in hindsight. All they knew was that I was retiring from climbing and moving to L.A., which seemed as dismissive as it was crazy. As much as I ask them to believe me, it's also my responsibility to understand their response. Accountability can come quickly but forgiveness can take time. Sometimes it never comes at all.

It's also my responsibility to listen to myself. I drive to U-Haul, buy twenty-five boxes and three rolls of packing tape, and try to guess how many books I have. Second chances are for everyone. Sometimes second chances are granted to us, by us.

And still, one more thing must fall away.

34

We are not mad, we are human. We want to love,

and someone must forgive us the paths we take to love,

for the paths are many and dark, and we are

ardent and cruel in our journey.

—Leonard Cohen

"Who's there?" Narcissus called out, aware that he was being watched. Echo was entranced by his beauty and had been spying on him from the forest. But Echo had been cursed to have no voice of her own. After she had distracted Hera from the affairs of Zeus, the goddess punished her by taking her words. She could only repeat the words spoken to her.

"Who's there?" Echo called back.

Echo wanted to love Narcissus but she couldn't communicate it. It would have been no use anyway. Narcissus was cursed to only love himself. After rejecting Echo, he drowned in a shallow pond when he fell in as he stared at his own reflection. Eventually his body was absorbed by the earth and he came back as a flower, unable to gaze upon its own beauty.

She's achingly beautiful and when I meet her, my mind is silent. The double helix of my DNA contracts and tangles itself around her. The shift is subatomic as all the cells of my body rearrange themselves into something so whole that the word *complete* is incomplete. I'm the best kind of crazy and believe in love songs that I've always hated. How could so much art be wrong?

She has a tiny, colorless mole above her eye and a scar from a bee sting that looks like a freckle. Perfectly disheveled strands of chocolate hair frame high cheekbones. She moves almost silently, and I notice her ankles and wrists. When she looks up from a book about psychopaths, she extends a delicate middle finger that says, "I love you. Stop looking at me." She's taken every word and rearranged the letters to spell her own, impossibly long word that is an adjective, noun, and verb in a thousand different languages. The word confuses me because there is no definition other than her, and I imagine my life leading directly to her doorstep. I need to understand that path and memorize it so I can always find my way back. If everything in my life has brought me here, I'd do it all again without hesitation, because for the first time I feel like I understand what home means.

When we make love, it's more energy than matter, and there is no space. There is no piece of her that I don't want as she pushes me away and says, "Get away, weirdo!" when I playfully smell her armpits. I'm greedy and want her sweat and her spit and her anger. I want her hand on my leg as we drive from somewhere to anywhere in silence. I don't care where we're going so long as it's together.

She helps me buy eight more boxes and we stack them in a truck. I sign a yellow piece of paper and watch them drive west as we climb into my car and I ask her to DJ. She sits next to me and I hear the tiny clicks of her phone and John Vincent III sings, "When you get tired of this town / Let me know, and we can go somewhere brand-new."

"This song always reminds me of you," she says without looking up. I feel my foot lean into the gas pedal and Colorado becomes my past.

We drive across the country toward a new life together and

make nude pictures of each other in big, lonely landscapes. They are some of the best, most creative images I've ever made. The lightness of it all allows me to share my darkness, and all my secrets seep out as we look at each other across pillows. We forgive everything about each other because being human is too complex to judge. Because she's a mirror of all my parts, I judge myself less when I look at her.

I tell her all my secrets of infidelities and lies and the shame that I hold on to. I tell her that I have used all the external validation of my life to mask an unrelenting fear of rejection. I say, "I've always hated my belly," and she says, "Me too," as she wraps her arms around me from behind and kisses my neck as we stare in a mirror in a cheap hotel in Nevada. I've learned to be weary of love because my brain has a habit of misguiding me. She tells me to "stop trying to figure it out." She tells me to trust and I do.

She's an artist but her talents have been overshadowed by her face, and quickly I see that her beauty is as much a curse as a blessing. I think it's a cruel irony that someone who everyone notices can feel so overlooked. She stops rooms and despite her talents, the world has taught her that her value is only skin-deep. That's where the money is.

Just after we met, I was empathizing with her over how hard it is to be a full-time artist even though I still rejected the label. She was uncharacteristically quiet and lowered her gaze and told me in short sentences that she works in a darker world, behind closed doors in rooms filled with cigar smoke and cocaine and rich men who wear expensive cologne that smells cheap. She sits on their laps and studies hidden hands of Texas Hold 'Em knowing that if the men win they'll slide thousands of dollars of chips to her or tuck them in the lingerie in too-familiar ways. This is *Molly's Game*, but for her it's no movie and it's no game at all. To the players she's a thing. To everyone she's a thing. An idea. A fantasy.

But the money is good, and she told me that by taking it from them, she felt like she could pull something back from what the world of men had taken from her. And it was a lot. I couldn't understand this, but it made me hurt. I promised that I'd never judge because my own secrets make judgment impossible. Where we are is where we've been. I hated the idea of what she did for work, but I also thought I could handle it. I promised to stand by her for as long as it took and said, "I can't save you. But I can be here." I didn't see it now, but I'll learn this was its own deceit.

A month later we're in my new apartment in L.A. and I can smell the ocean. She sits on the wood floor in front of the mirror and applies a delicate line of eyeliner before she slides into lingerie and asks, "How do I look?" The outfit isn't for me and my stomach aches. Before I can answer she says, "My Uber is here," kisses me, and slips out the door.

I stare at the ceiling and try not to imagine some random man's hand on her thigh. I can't sleep on these nights as I wait for her text telling me that she's safe. Instead, I wrestle with my imagination. All I can ask is that she tell me the truth, and she always says, "I am," with a hint of defensiveness. As much as I want to be strong enough to hold this space, it's driving a wedge between us.

It's 3:01 A.M. and I'm sitting in my car across the street from an obscure house in the Hollywood Hills. I feel gross, as if I'm somehow supporting this world I hate so much. A muscular security guard in black talks into a headset as she appears from a gate and crosses the road and gets in the car, a little drunk and playful. We drive home and she counts a thick pile of cash and I think it seems like a lot for just being pretty.

Another night she gets in the car in silence and cries and won't let me touch her. Two of the purest expressions of love are consistency and patience, and I strain for both as I sit quietly, listening to her sniffle. "I think we should get away for a while." It's an offer of escape and she puts her hand on my leg and agrees.

A week later, we pack the car and drive east through the Mojave listening to true-crime podcasts. She's an aficionado of the macabre and I've mapped out a string of haunted hotels to stay in. At night, we sneak through the halls taking nude pictures under blinking yellow lights that buzz above a red carpet with coffee stains and vacuum burns. In a cheap hotel in New Mexico where spaghetti Western stars used to stay, we lie in a pool of sweat and she asks, "Do you want to marry me?" It's a joke but not a joke. "More than anything," I reply. After two weeks, the space between us seems repaired and we drive home, hoping the sweetness will stay.

I make her an old-fashioned with a big spherical ice cube and watch little bursts of flame as I squeeze an orange peel into a lighter. I run the rind around the lip of the glass and take it into the living room, and we watch reruns while she falls asleep in my lap.

In the morning, I watch her dress and notice an increasing modesty as she turns away from me. She hates every picture I take of her, picking herself apart with relentless criticism.

We drive to Venice and dip into a store with a thousand tiny things that make a house a home. She hands me a small notepad with a faded blue cover and a pen and tells me to buy it.

"I have an idea." She smiles.

"Tell me."

"I'm going to pick a person or an object . . . anything . . . and you have to write a one-page story about it."

"Is this to shut me up so I stop asking questions?"

"That's a bonus, doofus. But no. I think you should write." After the fallout of my abrupt exit from climbing and the end of my work with *National Geographic,* my life has an unfamiliar formlessness to it. She can sense it, and I know that if I don't flex the muscles of creativity, they will slowly atrophy. I buy the pen and pad and follow her out into the sun.

"Are you hungry?"

"I could eat."

We step into Gjelina and sit at a high top and order pizza as she scans the room. For my first story, she picks a man with glasses, long hair, and salt-and-pepper stubble and says, "Him."

"Don't lie. It's because you think he's hot." She laughs and doesn't disagree. I begin to write and remember how much I love cursive. It's how I'll start this book.

Sweet days like this fill me up, but they seem to be fewer and farther between. I can sense that her excitement for us is fading and I mistake it for the waning of our honeymoon phase. Some days she's so silent that I can't hear anything but the place where her words used to be. I ask more questions and she answers with a word. Gradually, she stops laughing at my jokes. When I call her, she answers quietly and I overcompensate with cheerfulness, which makes her quieter. The silence at dinner makes me talk more. I wish I'd shut up and stop trying but instead try harder, reaching for something that feels like it's slipping away.

A few times I help her buy outfits that she'll wear for other men at the poker games. I wish she'd wear them for me like she used to. But now that she's safe, the lace is reserved for her job because the world of me and the world of work are incompatible.

I can't have the fantasy and the real at the same time. I'm also confused, because a piece of me likes being the person who sleeps next to the fantasy and I imagine myself as strong as I wrap around her. But this isn't strength no matter how much I want to believe it is.

Some nights she comes home from work smelling like cigars and the cologne that the men sweat onto her. Sometimes she wants to fuck. Other nights she won't let me touch her. I stare at the ceiling and wonder why. But then she rolls over and grabs my hand and I forget it all, exchanging the pain for a moment of connection. There is an escalating polarity in our relationship where my happiness relies on her happiness. For me to be okay, she has to be okay and I remember words like *co-dependent* and *toxic* and *enabling* but ignore them. Instead, I chip away little pieces of my own well-being, hoping that I can trade them for a smile or that she might hold my hand for a few moments longer before pulling away.

The more I bend into the shape of her, the more tension I feel because somehow I'm becoming invisible. But I don't have the words to tell her what I need and it traps her in my own silence. The fear of losing her makes me mute, and I wonder how anyone who talks as much as me can be so ineffective at communicating. I'm fighting for the attachment over authenticity because attachment is addictive and comfortable and sticky. I love her and I won't let go even though she's quietly asking me to.

Finally I feel that I might disappear altogether, and we begin to yell and criticize and fight and say things we don't mean. But the words don't really matter. We're just yelling to be seen. I feel childish and stupid. I feel crazy because none of this feels like me and I don't remember when I became an angry person. I pivot and correct for careless words and apologize for the wrong things until we come together again. I can't say what I need to say because I don't have the courage to lose her. What I need to say is, "None of this works."

It's been six months since I moved to California. After about a week of scribbling short stories about strangers, dogs, and coffee cups, the first pages of this book started spilling out. But now I'm stumped and distracted by L.A. I've never been stationary for this long. I've traveled nine months a year for the past decade and I'm beginning to feel trapped.

"Do you want to go away again?"

"You mean like to the desert?" She looks at me.

"No. Like far away. You can get away from poker and I can write and we can just get the fuck out of L.A." A piece of me wonders if all of the discomfort of our relationship might be erased under a different sky. It's the same reason people buy houses and make babies when they feel a partnership failing, creating something that they hope will irrevocably bond them. It rarely works.

She pauses before answering. "Okay. But I'm going to have to work a lot before we go." It sounds more like a question than a statement, as if she's asking if I'm okay with it. I'm not, but what can I say? If I want to stay with her, it's a trade I have to make.

The idea of moving momentarily pulls us back together, and we plot our escape to an island in Southeast Asia where dinner costs five dollars and we can stretch our savings for six months. There, there will be no more dark rooms and expensive cologne that smells cheap. Instead, we'll smell humid air and the sea, and I hope all the little pieces of me that I've surrendered to the relationship will be filled back in with salt and sun. I sell my car and pack all the boxes again and put them in storage, escaping to a fresh start and the promise of renewed love. We board the plane on New Year's Eve and watch the city fall away.

We land in a nearly abandoned Bangkok airport. People in

masks move around each other at a distance and flinch when anyone sneezes. After ramen for breakfast, we make our way to our next flight and sit in the boarding area. I don't know where it comes from, but it's here now, coming like an avalanche.

Truth is often known long before it's spoken, and I've known the truth before she tells me. Her words fall out like the last snowflakes before a slope collapses under its own weight and I think of all the avalanches of my life. There is loaded silence before they come and every muscle in my body contracts. By now I know that I can't outrun them and I wish the silence of my ignorance would suck the words back up before they bury me. But it's too late and what she tells me is something I always suspected.

I'm standing outside a window and I watch his hands on her as she closes the door and reaches for his belt and smiles at him the way she smiles at me after dinner. Now I am hovering above them on the bed and now I lie next to her and watch her face pushed down onto the mattress in a tangle of dark hair beneath knuckles and fingers and nails. Hands grasp. I listen to the sounds she makes and wonder what is real and what is a ghost and which memories are now dead. I feel her heart as she asks him to slap her hard across the face. I see his face twist as he stares down the depression of her spine, grabbing her waist and pulling her into him. Confusion and disdain and fear and disgust. Pleasure and power and detachment; a million mountains of entanglement spread across her skin as the goosebumps I've memorized. Every expression of emotion is accounted for. Aside from joy. There is no joy here and I watch it all, buried under a pile of crisp hundred-dollar bills that have been passed between hands.

She tells me what she has been hiding and I'm searching for judgment but find none. On other nights at other points in my life I have been him, exchanging money for sex and validation that I can touch but never feel. I watch the abused and the abuser as both and feel three expressions of pain—for her, for me, and for the times that I was the anonymous man thrusting himself into someone else's life—and I'm unable to turn away from the vision in my head. Seeing what I've done being done to the person I love most is unbearable and I don't understand what piece of it I hate most.

The digital numerals on the clock glow bright and blue. Her phone is lying facedown on the nightstand so my messages won't disrupt the emotional compartmentalization she needs. 3:17 A.M. I watch them until he collapses and kisses her spine. Kisses her forehead in feigned tenderness and says, "Thank you." And she says nothing.

Had I not been in that same room on different nights, this wouldn't be my story to tell. But I have and now this is our story and we are the same person reaching for each other in all the wrong ways. Of all the behaviors that come with bipolar, hypersexuality has been the one that I've struggled with most. I've paid for sex to feel "close" to someone, to feel in control of my life for a moment. But as soon as I'm walking back to my car smelling like a stranger, I'm more isolated, more out of control, and vacant. If the woman in the dark room on the fourth floor feels half of this, there is no apology that can ever suffice. This is us and this is me and staring at yourself can be a painful process and the boarding agent says, "It's now time to board flight 457 for your island future."

When we land, I buy a burnt chocolate croissant and two coffees. I'm not angry . . . that will come later. She's kept her promise and told the truth. I'm hurt that the truth was present as we packed the boxes. It was there, hidden under the conversation at Thanksgiving and Christmas. I'm confused that she could watch me surrender myself to a big, uncertain future with her while holding a secret that's been eating our love like a termite, the same way I had in my marriage. She knew that the truth might break us.

I understand why she couldn't tell me until this moment. It required her escape to feel safe enough. She needed to tell me in the space between our old life and new life because there, maybe, it could be forgiven; it might crash into the ocean that separated the two. She knows that I have my own past with this very thing, so as much as betrayal has a way of erasing the memory of our own transgressions, I am no saint. I've made many mistakes and told my own lies. She asks if I want to leave her. I don't. But it isn't a question. It's a request and she's not asking if I want to leave her. She's asking me to leave her.

We move into a white house high on a steep hill of tangled jungle. The white walls match the white floor and rise to the ceiling with an east-facing wall of glass that slides all the way open. We buy three large plants of various greens and one desert rose that blooms bright pink flowers and bakes in direct sun and drinks rainwater. We hang our clothes in the closets, and she chooses three images for the lifeless walls and the house inches toward being a home. We learn the aisles of a new grocery store and try to read labels in a language we don't understand. I learn to trap huge spiders that move impossibly fast while she pretends to dry-heave and we distract ourselves with everything new. We buy a hand-sewn rug and unroll it under the couch and hope it's big enough to hide all the shit we're trying to sweep out of sight. And still, it's clear that moving across the world is not going to fix the structural fissures in our relationship. If anything, it's slowly making them worse.

I try to write but nothing comes out because my mind is tied up with her and us and she seems to be moving as far away from me as we've moved away from home. I ask if she loves me.

"Of course," she says.

"Of course."

After a month, we're fighting more than we speak. We yell and slam doors and push through them and say things we don't mean. Cruelty is a language of pain. I want to blame it all on her but I know I can't. I agreed to this and in many ways enabled it in

hopes that I could in fact save her. But now, it's as if I'm a re-
minder of the darkness of her life back home and the last piece
she needs to shed before she can truly move on.

In truth, I've built a story of her and created beliefs around it.
When she doesn't live up to the expectations of my own fiction,
I'm somehow surprised. I'm judging her against an ideal I created
and ignoring what's real. And if I'm honest, I've buoyed myself to
her beauty, hoping that standing next to her might make me
valuable; hoping that external love might somehow make me
whole.

Six weeks after we land, we crumble. I lean against the wall
with my arms crossed and look at her. She twists and rests her
head on the back of the couch.

"Would you be happier without me?" I ask.

"Would you be happier without *me*?"

In love, the question is often the answer.

I drive her to a new neighborhood and a cozy beach bungalow
feet from the ocean and help decorate a living room I'll never live
in. There's a new rug for feet that will replace mine within a
month. A new chair to cradle a new body. Someone else to pour
her whiskey.

I install a new light fixture above a bed and imagine her making love to someone new. I connect the wires and turn the screwdriver and take care not to leave footprints on the sheets because
she hates mess. I hope when she turns the light on she'll see me.
As much as I want her to believe my kindness is maturity, it's just
another way to hold on.

She adopts an adorable, emaciated street dog named Olive
because she's tiny and black. I think maybe the dog can tie us
back together with chew toys and midnight potty breaks. Instead, Olive stops breathing early one morning as I cradle her.

We drive frantically to every vet on the island, but all the doors are locked as I listen to sobs I've never heard before and give CPR to a lifeless and limp puppy. I tried to save her. I tried to save them both. But then again, maybe I had always been trying to save myself from drowning in a pond.

After Olive dies, she closes the doors and shuts the blinds and pushes me away because the last sweet piece of our life together literally died in my arms. We become "was." I give away the pictures we'd hung and the plants and roll up the beautiful rug and put it in a box and ship it to California half hoping it will get lost in the mail. I want every day to end so I can forget while I sleep, but I can't sleep at all.

As real as the love felt, somehow, we'd fallen into the trap of co-dependence and it had made it impossible to grow. In relationship, our suffering is relative to the degree that we sacrifice ourselves. When I was present in her life, she didn't need to evolve because I would always "rescue" her. And she'd never asked for that.

Trying to save someone is an arrogant form of people-pleasing that hides selfishness behind care-taking. Often, that which we are trying to mend in another is just a mirror of where we see ourselves as broken. Hard as it might be to accept, trying to fix someone is deeply narcissistic behavior.

I'd given her all of my power and stolen all of hers because that's what "saving" a person does. It isn't respect. It isn't love. It's an arrogant extraction of agency. It does not say "I love you." It says, "You are a broken thing."

Two months after splitting up, I buy a ticket back to America and watch the island get swallowed by a thunderstorm. When my plane lands in L.A., I have three bags with stubborn sand stuck in the bottom and I begin to reimagine my definitions of "home" and "complete" and for months she haunts me in twelve-hour intervals. Once at 3:30 in the morning, when I see her wrapped in sun and sweat and skin, in love with someone new, separated by an ocean, I bury my face in the pillow and scream. And then again at 3:30 in the afternoon when all the anger is exhausted and all I can do is miss her. Smiling hurts.

Eventually I move into a 200-square-foot apartment so there is no room for anyone else and it will be harder to lose pieces of myself. There is comfort in the smallness because I can't condense any further and my only choice is growth. I'm angry until I'm not and realize that we're lucky if we get one person who can teach us so much, no matter how flawed that love might be. Another person can never make us whole, but they can inspire us to change. I think of Narcissus and Echo again and hear Kamila Shamsie's words: "People don't change." "People change entirely," I said. "Look at Narcissus. Became a flower. I call that change."

In losing her, the last source of external value I can cling to is finally stripped away. She led me to the precipice of lasting change that I didn't know I needed to make. She led me back to myself.

35

Never miss a good chance to shut up.

—WILL ROGERS

A bell rings and I open my eyes to darkness and study the soft blur of a mosquito net over my bed. It hangs from plywood walls and drapes in translucent white wrinkles, tied to the four tiny nails that keep it suspended above my body like a gossamer cage. The room is roughly 4 by 8 feet with the bed tucked in the back right corner, propped 3 feet off the ground on two-by-fours, under a glassless window with four bars painted white. I'm thirty-nine years old. What is foreign is now more *home* than home and I wonder for the nth time what the word means or if there is a definition at all.

The bell rings again and comes in rhythmic intervals, starting softly and building throughout thirty-three versions of itself and I wonder how many versions of myself I've been. I resist the instinct to look at my watch or phone until I remember I have neither because I tied them in a bag and surrendered them the day before. But I already know the time. It's 4:30 A.M.

I've woken so many times to strange rooms on foreign soil that the experience no longer surprises me. The haphazard symphony of jungle sounds buzzing and whining and screeching and chirping and singing in the blue shadows outside sing the national anthem of Thailand. The first lesson of silence is that the world is a very loud place.

I stare down the lines of my naked body, stretched out on a single grass mat insulating me from a plywood slat. I'm calling this a "bed," which seems like a pretty generous term. "Monk's pillow" is even more generous. A single block of wood nine inches wide and four inches thick props my skull, demanding that I sleep on my back or side. A gentle cutout cradles my head as much as a wood pillow can cradle anything. A thin blanket is cast aside in a dark clump at my feet.

I roll to my side to sit up and feel bruises on my hips from the hard platform and wince. I pull the mosquito net from under the mat where I tuck it every night before staring at the ceiling and trying to sleep. I tuck it in to keep the ants and mosquitoes and spiders and lizards and bats from interrupting my already fragile rest. I think of Mom, who never sleeps as much as stares at the backside of her eyelids, still listening for me to come home thirty-nine years later.

Yesterday my 125 cc scooter whines and hums as I drive up a road that would be illegal in most parts of the world. The slope is at least 27°, 32° in places, and threatens to throw the front tire into a wheelie when I throttle down. But on the islands in the gulf of Thailand, a "road" is just a slick of concrete poured down a hill, as much as a "bed" is just a piece of plywood.

The asphalt switches back once, then again before gaining the spine of ridge and the world falls away on both sides. I feel the cool, humid air against my skin, rising up from the sea 1,200 feet below.

I park and wander into a large open-sided building with a peaked fiberglass roof and tile flooring and sit in front of a man who never looks at me and stares at the floor as if his eyes might fall from their sockets and I wonder if a person can meditate too much. He talks in a slow German drawl verging on slurring and explains the guidelines of my residency, a so-called Vipassana hermitage.

No reading.

No writing.

No electronics.

No cigarettes.

No drugs.

Don't jerk off.

Do not kill anything.

Adhere to the schedule.

Do my chores.

And above all, *never, ever* speak with fellow participants. I pretend to zip my lips and flick the key into the air. He doesn't smile.

I think about all the languages I've heard and spoken and wonder how language is born and how it dies. Pali, a dead language of the Indian subcontinent, is believed to be the language of a man named Siddhartha Gautama. His more common name is the Buddha.

Vipassana is a Pali word translated as "insight." Other translations include "clear seeing" or "great vision." You get the picture.

At its core, Vipassana is a meditation practice that seeks insight through breathing. Breathing is the first thing we are given and the last thing that's going to leave. We can always find it and, in time, learn to follow it. And if we're vigilant the nature of everything will be revealed. That's it . . . just follow your breath to enlightenment. Easy!

But because it's always with me, I've grown deaf to the constant rhythm of my breath, exchanging awareness for thought, and I learn the second lesson of silence: My brain is really, *really* loud. I've always known this but by silencing myself I'm hearing the noise more clearly and growing increasingly aware of its incessant and unending barrage of mostly useless thoughts.

Some science suggests we have about sixty thousand thoughts a day, 95 percent of which are repeated. Of those, roughly 80 percent are negative. Amidst those negative thoughts, we spend roughly 160 hours a year worrying. We often imagine and *live* hypothetical realities, dredging up all the terrible emotions that come with them. But roughly 85 percent of this menagerie of doom *never happens.* Just 15 percent of our miserable fictions ever come to pass. Not all thoughts become reality. In fact, very few do. It's the stories they reinforce and the emotions they ignite that are real. And yet despite all the clatter the brain is only capable of one thought at a time. Just one.

But the brain is really fast. The speed of thought is quantified in different measures, from bits (11 million per second) to land speed (if they were let out of their cage, some thoughts could travel 393.6 feet per second) and I hear Dad doing all the calculations. My thoughts can move twice as fast as the avalanche that almost stole my breath and all my thoughts eleven years ago.

These numbers race through my mind and it feels a lot like mania. I'm not manic, but thirteen minutes into a week of silence my history with "racing thoughts" blurs into something altogether more terrifying: the dumpster fire of consciousness.

Dizzyingly, *all* of these thoughts flood my brain while I am still sitting in front of the big-eyed German. I sign my name on a piece of paper and move to a chair in front of a silent lady with straight salt-and-pepper hair and fair Asian skin with fine wrinkles. She takes my things and ties them in a cotton bag and assigns me a number and hands me a different bag. In it is the blanket and mosquito net. She slides another piece of paper in front of me with a list of chores to choose from.

"Sweep the path from the meditation hall to the women's dorm" is perfect because I find sweeping very satisfying and maybe I'll get to smile at the cute girl with dark hair and tattoos.

I write my name in meticulous block letters in the space opposite the assignment and gather my duffel full of loose-fitting clothes and bedding and walk up another steep road to an open-sided building. The bottom floor is dug into the hillside and is a small maze of white plywood "rooms" that remind me of cells, each with a wooden pillow and grass mat. None of the doors close without being forced. None of the windows are covered. The ceiling hangs low and dark above me and I notice large spiderwebs, undisturbed because this is their home more than mine.

I walk past one of the empty rooms and see two fist-sized holes in an empty bed and remember every night I've ever spent in psychiatric hospitals and rehabs and wonder who made the holes and what it looked like when he did. What did it sound like? Did he scream? Did he break the bones in his hands punching through the platform? Was there blood? Was it the silence or his own thoughts that drove him mad? Can they be separated? What were his first words after he broke his silence? Where is he now? What is he doing? I'm alarmed at the speed with which I imagine all these things. Nine unanswerable questions in the span of two steps. A flood of emotion and imagined things that happened but no longer exist. A story.

I find an empty room and hang the mosquito net and lie down on the bed to feel how hard it really is. I rest my head on the wooden wedge and think it looks a bit like medieval blocks used for decapitation. The guillotine was last used in 1977 and I think that is a much more effective means of ridding the mind of thought.

My schedule for the next week is a reduction to the most basic acts of living. After I wake at 4:30 A.M., the seventeen-hour days will unfold in a rhythm of ten hours of meditation, interrupted by two meals, chores, instruction on the practice, and three hours of free time to wonder what the fuck I'm doing here.

As the days progress, I learn the third through tenth lessons of silence. They are as follows:

3. I'm going to go crazy
4. I'm going crazy
5. I'm crazy
6. Crazy
7. Brazy
8. Breazy
9. Breathe
10.

The lessons of silence will repeat moment by moment, hour by hour, and day by day. I'll go crazy and find my breath several times in a minute. And when I think I've cleared my mind and the thoughts disappear, I'll feel pride and accomplishment, which inevitably sends my brain catapulting back into a shitstorm of more thought. It happens over and over and over until the repetition itself makes me crazy and I come back to my breath again and relearn that meditation is not about clearing your mind as much as it's about noticing the thoughts, watching them, and letting them pass like clouds. When we start, our mind is overcast. But over time, with enough repetition, the storm begins to clear.

No mountain or assignment or expedition has ever been this difficult to manage. As much as activities like climbing and photography create a sense of presence, they feed thought and problem-solving, whereas silence and the simple activity of observation lay my mind bare and the only problem-solving is how to make it all stop. But when I try to make it stop, I'm already thinking.

Meditation comes in a myriad of forms, from Vipassana to Transcendental and Vedic (mantra meditation) to Yoga Nidra. Meditation isn't necessarily a religious practice and it's not tied to faith, though you might end up feeling more spiritual.

The benefits of meditation have been widely studied and, unsurprisingly, all the findings support what ancient wisdom has been saying for eons. But what the sages of the past could only observe, science can prove. So, here you go: Among the documented scientific findings, meditation reduces cortisol and inflammatory chemicals called cytokines, which amplify symptoms of anxiety and depression, raise blood pressure, and cause brain fog. It reduces the inflammation response of stress and strong evidence suggests that it can improve symptoms of a wide variety of stress-related conditions, from irritable bowel syndrome to PTSD. It provides positive shifts in anxiety, pain (emotional and physical), and depression. It enhances self-awareness as we begin to recognize our emotional patterns. Once we see them more clearly, the road is opened to change. In this way, meditation has been shown to increase impulse control by identifying triggers that promote addictive behaviors.

Similarly, self-awareness can help us be more empathetic and improves self-efficacy. One study showed that feelings of loneliness were reduced after just two weeks of daily meditation. It also builds our attention span and may even reverse patterns of rumination and worry. Evidence suggests it can reduce memory loss as we get older. A meta-analysis of twenty-two studies on loving-kindness meditation, also called Metta, proved its ability to increase compassion, both toward ourselves and toward others. So it's safe to say meditation is pretty good for us. You can do it anywhere at any time. Here, I'll show you:

Put down the book, set a timer on your phone for one minute, close your eyes, and follow your breath. You're going to think. Don't worry. Just notice yourself think. Notice yourself thinking about thinking. And just come back to the breath.

There. You just meditated. Congratulations. You didn't betray God and you didn't levitate and you did it "right," I promise.

You don't need to go into silence on a hill in a jungle and sweep until you lose your mind. You don't have to meditate for an hour a day. And trust me when I say this: There is no "wrong" meditation. If someone is selling you "the best way to meditate," walk away. Do what works for you. Try all the methods. Play with it. If something doesn't work, don't do it. There is no such thing as a bad meditation, just like there is no such thing as a bad day at the gym. Your brain might be all over the place, but you still showed up, and now I'm opening my eyes and thinking, "Holy shit . . . I don't think I followed one whole breath!" It happens all the time. What's most important with meditation is consistency. Start really small. Start with thirty seconds, if that's what you've got. That's enough. Just keep doing it. Did you miss a day? Me too. All the time. Shit, I've missed six months. That's okay. It only takes one day to start and you didn't throw away the progress because you fell off the wagon. Meditation is for life. Oh, and by the way, did I mention it's free?

Meditation offers the opportunity to see things as they are. Once you're there, change happens. For a moment, stop trying. Just feel what it is to be you.

On day one I glide across the floors on my tiptoes, mindful of all the sounds my body makes. I make a game of it, feeling my feet land and observing anything I hear. When I touch a bowl or a cup or my toothbrush, I notice the pressure of my hands and textures of the objects. When I eat, I count the number of times I chew, trying to get to twenty before swallowing. It's a technique I learned in a mindful-eating class in rehab as an addict's method to slow shoving food where the booze or smoke or pills used to go. I notice the softness and temperature of the polished floor of the meditation hall and the unforgiving, cold resistance of tile. The first day passes easily because my brain is immersed in a stimulating new game and I'm probably already enlightened because I'm just so fucking good at noticing everything. Just wait.

On day two the bell rings again and I sit up and touch the

mosquito net with renewed attention before forgetting to notice anything and rushing to the showers. The cold water splashes across my body and my breath is short and labored as I try to adjust the temperature, noticing the resistance of the knob and the texture of the metal. But there is only one temperature: cold. So I lather myself in a thick film of cheap soap that smells like chemical flowers and stand under confronting LED lights that cast shadows in all the wrong places. My skin is all goosebumps as I notice more spiderwebs and dried urine on the toilet seat. I lose my focus as I rinse off and won't follow another breath for hours.

After breakfast, I grab a bamboo staff with stiff sticks lashed around the bottom. As with so many things here, the label "broom" seems generous.

The path I'm meant to sweep is a collection of steep, narrow cement stairs, breeze-block pathways, and sand that winds its way through the forest. The rain from the previous day has flattened thousands of leaves against the pavement like stickers and the harder I sweep the stickier they become. Over the course of the week I'll learn that a gentle hand lifts the pasty leaves with ease, but that will take time.

Where there's breeze block, hundreds of leaves sit lodged in the holes, stubbornly out of reach of my sticks. When people walk by, I stand to the side of the pathway and look at the ground hoping they notice how vigilant I am in my silence. It occurs to me that even now, when I can't tell anyone about who I am and what I've seen and all my opinions, even the act of sweeping is an attempt to be acknowledged.

Day three comes too early, but I'm already awake, massaging the bruises on my hip bones and skull, craving a cigarette and food that isn't rice. I notice the cold water in the shower, but only because it annoys me. Wet and shivering, I stand impatiently behind shirtless men as they brush their teeth over concrete sinks. I hear their spit and gargling and farts and the urge to stab someone with my toothbrush makes me study the tall blond guy to my left, scanning his neck for the carotid artery. He's vascular and handsome and is probably my past lover's future boyfriend. Almost certainly. I'll need to sharpen my toothbrush into a shiv after sweeping.

At breakfast I forget to chew altogether and imagine writing a horror script about a silent retreat that goes terribly, terribly wrong. After winning an Oscar, I sweep the stairs harder, sweat three liters, and get lost.

I feel like a cynical version of Elizabeth Gilbert in *Eat Pray Love*. I'm very hungry. My singular prayer is that this ends before my mind melts. And love is . . . well, love is something but I have no idea what. Regardless, I understand the immense privilege of being able to take a week out of my life and sit in silence but question why anyone, anywhere, at any time would do such a thing to themselves. I hope that a blue light will shoot out of the top of my head in a metaphysical awakening. It won't.

When my window of free time comes in the afternoon, I feel a compulsive urge to sweep the pathway again. I'm sleep-deprived but I don't feel tired. So, I make my way up the stairs and start to feel the ground under my feet again. And when the first motion of the bristles hits my ears, I begin to notice *everything*, like the world is new. Or maybe someone spiked the tea with LSD. It's hard to know.

The first thing I see are thousands of tiny yellow star-shaped flowers that line the pathways. Next are the fluorescent pink leaves that I've somehow never seen because I've been walking around staring at my feet. There are thin, yawning leaves of dark green that have vibrant yellow splashes across them. Then sprouted coconuts. Then great vines wrapping themselves up the trunks of even bigger trees. Then the thousands of ants that attack my feet and broom. Then the smell of wet dirt. The white sky peeking through the canopy. The tiny bird to my right. The sound of a falling leaf. The sound as it hits the ground. The sound of the jungle whistling and screeching and ticking and buzzing. *Everything*. It's as if I'm waking up from a long, busy sleep. I feel a sense of awe for everything except the mosquitoes . . . I don't feel awe for them. Because fuck mosquitoes. And still I don't kill any.

On day four I break my vow of silence and whisper to a staff member, "May I buy some mosquito repellent?" as I scratch a quarter-sized bite on my left ass cheek. She shakes her head but says nothing. I spend 80 baht and retreat back into silence.

In my morning meditation something inside of me shifts. The old monk who talks about the possible experiences of meditation has described a deep sense of calm and a stillness that breaks through to insight and a brief sense of understanding about the nature of all things. What I experience isn't that but something equally as marvelous.

It starts slowly as I walk from the meditation hall to lunch. When I sit down to eat, the food appears as a mixture of everything that was required to bring it to the table. I imagine all the land, dirt, sun, and water needed to grow a leaf or a single grain of rice. I imagine all the cells inside a potato that have been cared for as they've grown and were pulled from the soil. I see dirt in the wrinkles of hands that dig and plant and harvest. I see the death and decay of the plants that came before them, relinquishing one existence for another before being plucked up as something new. People drive machines and fix water systems. They crate, bag, and box the food and place it on trucks and ships and planes, which are created by other people with big, brilliant brains. I see minerals dredged from the earth to make steel and aluminum and iron and watch people melt it down and pour it into forms that make the machines that move it all across the world. I marvel that the chair I sit in is made of materials that required thousands of minds to perfect before becoming an instrument of my comfort. The rivets on the table, fastening the legs to the plank. The material of the tiles and the hands that laid them on the floor. The trees that become the skeleton of the building. The corrugated roof that keeps the rain and sun off the tables. The bowl that holds the food and the spoon and the water in the glass.

Eventually it all leads back to a parade of every picture I've ever made flashing behind my eyes as everything I can see becomes worthy of gratitude. It's a feeling I've forgotten. And as nuts as it sounds, I can see one big, infinite cycle coming together as a single bite of food. For the second time in my life, the word *complete* is incomplete.

As it begins to overwhelm me I feel a bit batshit-crazy. But what's crazy isn't the recognition that so much is worthy of gratitude. What's crazy is that I haven't noticed it before as I replay my life in fast-forward, thinking of everything that moved me, fed me, and shaped me and I see how fortunate I have been. Being here at all is a display of my good fortune. I've been lucky not only to see the world but to continue to expand myself by changing my lens. A guy goes into a short, spiritual exile halfway around the world and wakes up: It's a humorous trope and I'm not blind to it.

But it's not just the privilege of who I am and what I've been able to do. Likewise, the revelation is accessible to anyone at any time, and how they come to it isn't really the point. It's the privilege of living at all, and this is a privilege we *all* share despite how hard life can be at times. The duality of our sorrows and joys is the buy-in. That I have a body that lives and breathes and moves is a gift. I have a body and mind that *gets* to be depressed, that *gets* to navigate ceaseless thought, and that has blood for a mosquito to steal, leaving me with enormous itchy welts.

I know it's easy to say something like that when you're sitting on a hill outside of the tempests of life. I know it's tragic that I've missed it and I know it's a cliché, but clichés have an annoying habit of being true. I laugh to myself and wonder if everyone here is as batshit as me. Maybe they think I'm crazy. Maybe I really am mad. Maybe being mad is okay. Maybe being mad is just being human.

On day six I'm on my hands and knees studying the transparent skin of a caterpillar. A collection of people scattered nearby are behaving equally as strangely. One has both hands on an enormous boulder, caressing it like a lover. A woman is standing a foot away from a concrete wall, staring at the cracks. Several more people are walking painfully slowly, breaking their steps into five distinct motions while staring intently at their feet, and I wonder if I'm in another psychiatric unit. I look over my shoulders for the orderlies in white sneakers and scrubs coming to feed us the pills and take us back inside. But they aren't there. Just more people moving in slow motion.

After lunch the silence becomes oppressive and I search for new paths to sweep, eventually veering off the cement to an open swath of sand through the trees. I've watched people all over the world sweep dirt roads, paths, and doorsteps that are made of the same dirt they're sweeping away and wondered why they do it. But I begin to understand. In its total futility, sweeping sand is one of the most gratifying experiences of my life, momentarily creating order from chaos.

After a long, muggy hour I'm staring at the sand, lost in thought, and I remember referring to my life as an hourglass with a single grain hanging in the neck—a single experience influenced by everything that came before and informing everything since. A moment when I almost lost my breath. I know I'm not *supposed* to be thinking, but I'm thinking a lot and wonder what pieces of me are worth keeping.

The etymology of *identity* is from the Latin *idem* and means "the same." It comes from *id*, "it," "that one." In the 1600s it became *identity*, which means "sameness" and "oneness" and "the state of being the same." You are the one, the same, because that's what you are. Identity begins with "I."

One of the central tenets of Vipassana (as an extension of Buddhism) is that everything we perceive is transient, constantly changing, and thus has no real identity. It's *our* identity and the mind's need to make order from chaos that form the reality we see. The leading edge of physics and quantum mechanics supports this. Atoms are exchanging and moving and shedding and nothing really is as we see it. To make it even more confusing, observing something changes its very nature.

Ninety-eight percent of the atoms that constitute our physical form are exchanged every year, replaced by particles that have lived a trillion lives. Gas. Liquid. Solid. Dinosaur. We are literally matter changing form every moment of every day. By that measure I'm not the same person as the person who started this sentence. Likewise, the cells that make up our bodies are replaced every seven to ten years. Ironically, the meat suit we're all wearing that we understand as the consistent "self" is not solid at all. We experience ourselves as constant but are anything but. We attach an identity to ourselves and everything else and hold on for dear life, often kicking and screaming when everything we thought was so solid changes.

Consistent meditation offers the opportunity to peel ourselves back from everything we're holding on to. With that distance, we can reexamine all the beliefs that shape us and now I'm thinking about being a "climber" and being a "photographer" and being "me." All the things I've anchored myself to are just ways to form an identity that is far more flexible than I'd like to believe. Letting go of it all is painful work.

My back is hunched and my legs are spread out in front of me.

I look like a five-year-old in a sandbox. I squeeze fistfuls of sand and my hands always end up empty. We can't hold on to anything forever.

The quieter I've become, the less certain of me I am. If I let go of all the words I've used to define me, who will I be? It feels like I'm sitting on the edge of some big realization and leaving a million pieces of me behind like the little piles of sand between my legs. But just as the sentiment crests, a searing red pain shoots through my body as an army ant sinks its enormous serrated mandibles into my crotch. I break my vows of silence and non-violence and vengefully squeeze the ant between my thumb and forefinger and say "Fuck!" a little too loud. For all the insight in the world, I'd never take back the murder. And so enlightenment evades me.

I wake up on the last day and the bell rings. Everyone begins to whisper as if they're making sure they still have a voice and I wonder who everyone "is." The cute girl with tattoos left early, so I have no one to flirt with and I sit drinking tea, wondering where I go from here. Something feels lighter, gone, new, and a little tender, like a snake shedding its skin as it eats its own tail.

I will turn forty next month. In the past two years I've left my job as a photographer, my father is dying, I've stopped climbing mountains, and I had to walk away from love. Somehow, despite it all, it's the most hopeful moment of my life and I think it's strange how fickle identity really is. Sometimes you have to shut up to hear yourself. I got everything I ever wanted and became someone I never wanted to be. Everything I've done is valuable, but it's not who I am. Not anymore.

The scooter tips down the steep road and the brakes squeal. I stop and smoke a cigarette because apparently nicotine is resistant to quantum physics. It tastes like it always does, burnt and bitter and a little disgusting, but I'm focused on the jungle and wondering how many things are changing form in front of me. I wonder, exactly in this moment, what comes next.

36

Words are, in my not-so-humble opinion,

our most inexhaustible source of magic. Capable of

both inflicting injury and remedying it.

—ALBUS DUMBLEDORE, in the film *Harry Potter
and the Deathly Hallows: Part 2*

"Do you want the front seat?" Dad is being chivalrous.

"No. I like the back."

"You sure? I'm happy to be in back."

"Yes."

"Guys, I think we've settled this one." I smile. This is a conversation we've had every morning for two weeks.

After Dhaulagiri, leaving both my jobs, moving to L.A., then Southeast Asia, then back to L.A., a broad space emerged between my parents and me. I'd call, but there was always a palpable tension. Dad and I spoke occasionally and I always felt guilty that I didn't have more to say. I haven't seen him in a year and a half. The doctors tell us he has four to six months left.

Today I wheel him through the Sistine Chapel and he cries. I'm sure it has something to do with Michelangelo. But more than that, I think it's about the toll that age extracts. He cries because he can barely walk. He cries because he feels like a burden. He cries because of the tender smiles we get, mostly directed at me, as we weave through the crowds of people who have all come to marvel at the house that faith built. Say what you want about religion—the art that has spilled from it is enough to make anyone stand in awe. I park the wheelchair and stand back as he looks up at paintings and sculptures and film his wonder and isolation. For Dad, time is racing toward its end and he can literally feel it in his joints. To lighten the mood, he asks if we should challenge another person in a wheelchair to a race. They decline. Probably for the best.

We spend our days in the car and Mom asks me, "How much longer?" while Dad tracks our progress on an eight-year-old GPS. He tells me to turn right when he means left and I follow Google Maps instead. The days have been long, humorous plays of shapeshifting from parent to child until we're all confused who is who.

"Mom, do you have snacks? Are you warm enough? What's your favorite movie?" *The Man from Snowy River.*

"Dad, you look like an unmade bed. How's the sciatica? Do you have your painkillers and an extra pair of underwear?" *The Lion in Winter.*

"Who wants gelato? Do they have salted caramel and *limone*? How many scoops? Cone or cup? What's one thing you would've told your parents before they died?" They both pause before Mom fills in the blank: "Please, just accept me for who I am rather than measuring me against who you wanted me to be."

We sit in a small courtyard and celebrate their fiftieth anniversary and I think how lucky I am to have them. I drink a glass of red wine in small sips. After six years of sobriety, I abandoned my identity as an addict. I don't advocate that for everyone, but it was one of a thousand stories I no longer needed; escaping excess for moderation was a long road that I simply took one day at a time.

After two weeks, the most time we've spent together since I left at fifteen, I pull the bags from the car and hand Dad the ski poles he needs to walk, and we enter the chaos of the airport. People move past us without noticing him as he hobbles on a drop foot and a hip that shifts in its socket. The airline attendants usher my parents to the front of the line and call for a wheelchair. Dad's fragility makes him appear still and isolated in a sea of blur. It's strange how the old can look so innocent after living a full life. He uses his thumb to wipe his cheeks. Whether he's crying from frustration that his body can't keep up with his mind or because we're saying goodbye, I can't tell.

I start walking to another terminal to catch my flight and I'm immediately bothered. Something doesn't feel right. I pat my pockets for my phone and passport. I look in my pack for my laptop and wallet. Something is missing but nothing is. *Do I need to pee? Why am I hot? My chest hurts. Whose hands are these?* I turn around and walk back and hope that Mom hasn't wheeled Dad off to their gate. I see the gentle hunch of his back through the crowd and slide in between the people stacked like sardines. The tops of his shoulders push through his shirt and I feel how thin his skin is as I slide my hand across his back.

I pull him into me as hard as I can and hold on. Mom watches us and I catch her eyes. As much as this book is a love letter to Dad, she's always been the backbone of our family and we've learned to talk without speaking. I need to say less to her because she knows. Moms do.

I pull back from Dad and bend a bit to be level with his eyes. I would say "I love you," but he knows. I would say "Go gently," but that's his. Instead, I just tell him he's a good dad. It sounds clunky and lacks all the poetry of Hollywood goodbyes. But it feels like this might be the last time I get to say anything and maybe it's something a father might like to hear.

Back in California, my hair is still a bit wet from the ocean and I feel sand against my scalp. Sometimes I don't shower after swimming because I like the smell of kelp and the way the salt feels on my skin. Sometimes I leave dishes in the sink and forget to brush my teeth too. As much as I have a flair for finding poetry in everything, I have no poetic reason for this.

I live in an old Spanish-style apartment on a street with tall palm trees that lean toward the Pacific and I can smell the sea most mornings. I stand in the kitchen, turn off the stove, ladle some bean stew into a bowl, and notice a beer stein from Salzburg. The small living room is full of books with coffee stains, dog-eared pages, and faded underlining. The books feel like they were written just for me, just like the lyrics I keep in my head. That's the beauty of art: it's for everyone.

There's a carved wooden bench I brought home from Nepal and a rug from Thailand and another from Iran. An old tea table from China with photo books stacked on top sits in front of a small couch. A writing desk is tucked in a nook with windows that face west.

A small crucifix from Mexico faces a page of an antique Quran from Pakistan. It hangs next to a small Buddhist statue from Mustang sitting on the mantel. A Tibetan belt buckle from the 1800s with a swastika in the middle reminds me that even the most beautiful stories and symbols can be twisted into something ugly. A Tibetan chest covered in faded paintings sits on the floor with a small piece of Marko's rib from Peru tucked behind a pair of goggles my great-uncle took to Everest before I was born. It's a house of stories.

I set the bowl on the bed because I have no dining table and lie down. I open my laptop and eat my stew as Harry Potter stands in some spiritual equilibrium, deciding whether or not to return to the living world. Harry asks Dumbledore, "Is this all real? Or is it just happening inside my head?"

Dumbledore replies, "Of course it's happening inside your head, Harry. Why should that mean that it's not real?"

———

The morning is dark when I wake up and the laptop is still open. The house is a bit chilly because I like to sleep with the windows open and I notice my nakedness in the mirror. The upstairs neighbors are having sex and I'm a bit jealous and wonder if they got up to brush their teeth or if they chose to be more honest and taste each other's sleep.

I pull on a sweatshirt and soft pants and feel my feet on the wood floor. A pillow rests on the floor in the living room and I sit, wrap a blanket around my shoulders, and close my eyes. At some point meditation stopped being a mind game. I've found that stillness is always accessible in that ineffable place in our chest. We quiet the mind to let the heart speak. When the heart listens, we use the mind to make sense of what it's heard. When a bell dings an hour later, I open my eyes. It's light outside, but the sun seems like it may be staying in bed today.

I heat up more bean stew and the radio is on. The politician or priest or whomever on the news reads a quote:

> Our Earth is degenerate in these later days; there are signs that the world is speedily coming to an end; bribery and corruption are common; children no longer obey their parents; every man wants to write a book and the end of the world is evidently approaching.

These aren't words from our times. Their provenance is dubious, but they're claimed to be inscribed on a clay tablet that predates Jesus by 2,800 years. Regardless, the point is clear: Humans have always thought we're living in the end-times. We've always been focused on death. Life's duality is the original black and white.

Storytelling is what we use to navigate life as well as transcend death. Story is consciousness. It drives discovery and belief and even psychology and science as we try to figure out and explain the why of things. Story is also the architecture of identity. We become "I" and the stories we tell ourselves not only guide us but become us. We say "I am this" and "You are that" and become certain of far too much. Story is the bedrock of everything we do and all the relationships we have. With others. With the world around us. With ourselves. Make no mistake, *storytelling is the most important thing we do.* To tell stories is to be human.

These days, the story of mental health has come into sharp focus as we try to normalize and understand its hurdles. I've played an active role in that and for the most part I think it's a positive shift. It's also important that we don't psychologize everything and everyone. In the new era of social media, the discussion around mental health has led to a sort of pathological self-obsession.

On a personal level, stories of mental health run deep and can be painfully confused with ideas of inadequacy and brokenness. Once we learn there is something "wrong" with us, it's easy to craft an identity around that and believe that we're fundamentally flawed.

As mental health has stepped into the forefront and the awareness around trauma has exploded, there also seems to be an unsustainable oversensitivity to anything personally bothersome, as if individuals are asking the world to walk on eggshells around their specific histories and triggers. This isn't realistic. Much as we might want society to adapt for our sensitivities, it's not everyone else's responsibility to accommodate our unresolved trauma. It's our responsibility to heal it. Psychology is an invitation out of victimhood, not into it.

I've spent most of my life trying to escape my own story of madness. I've chased the horizon, confusing it for a perfect future where everything will make sense. I've feared being myself because I learned early on that my mind was a dangerous thing. But in the pursuit of an idyllic version of me, I've missed the joy of being myself. Chasing the horizon is never wrong so long as we understand that, from another perspective, we're already there. I chose to live madly to outrun madness itself. I've thought that by rebellion, doing more, being better, and being different, I might be able to out-climb, out-explore, or out-create the disquiet of my mind. But what if the noise and madness were the gift?

Most mornings I read memoir. Some mornings I read about the brain. Sometimes I read fiction. This morning I'm reading *No Cure for Being Human* by Kate Bowler, who writes:

> I had nothing to do but survive the feeling that some pain is for no reason at all. It became clearer than ever that life is not a series of choices. So often the experiences that define us are the ones that we didn't pick. Cancer. Betrayal. Miscarriage. Job loss. Mental illness. A novel coronavirus.

Of all the things we can't choose, our personal story is one thing we can.

By saying you can choose a story, I'm not suggesting that provable facts and science are up for grabs. It's *your* story that you get to choose, not whether the earth is round or if climate change is real. I'm also not claiming that believing you don't have cancer or bipolar will cure it. There are far more people who have died of cancer and lived whole lives with mental illness than have cured themselves through positive thinking. To suggest these people endured and died because they didn't believe hard enough is, simply put, arrogant and cruel. Denial does not change basic facts. The brain can heal the body, no doubt, and positive thinking and psychology have real benefits. But sometimes things just are. Choosing our story is about stepping back and examining our thoughts and beliefs honestly. From that authenticity, we're invited to reframe the narrative of the journey.

In regard to mental illness, once we learn of our wounding, it's easy to make that the cornerstone of our identity and even hide behind it. By doing so, we become a victim. If I'm honest, I began this book from a place of victimhood. I was in my story so deep that I just couldn't see it. I'd pulled a blanket over my eyes but all the darkness did was hide the truth. I don't deny victimhood but it's only useful to emancipate ourselves from the pain of trauma. If we stay in the story too long, it becomes a cage. In time, even being a "survivor" can become an identity that keeps us anchored to the past. I was a victim for far too long.

I know how seductive holding on to suffering can be because I've done it. In many ways it feels safe. I know how powerful the identity of brokenness can be and I have many versions of this story. In one I have a flawed mind that I desperately need to repair. In another I'm beyond redemption, full of wicked behaviors and pathologies that hurt people. In this story I hang on to all my mistakes and shame. In one my brokenness fuels my creativity and I need to be tortured to create. In yet another I'm a burden, isolated outside a world that I can see but never touch. I have told and lived all these stories.

The story of my life, brain, and heart I choose now is this: I have a beautiful mind that is unique and wildly creative. It can be a bit temperamental at times. It developed to survive, and in survival I've thrived. It's driven me to make beautiful things and see the world. I'm not powerless to my sensitivity. My sensitivity gives me power. I embrace my mind even when it's messy. More and more, my heart guides the ship. It's not a story of unrealistic expectations of happiness or perfection. If I'm mindful, my polarity can be my depth. It has given me more middle to explore. I offer this story to everyone.

I'm sitting at my desk now and a small placard says "Do Epic Shit." I'm quite certain the sun has called in sick as I watch my fingers tap the little symbols and words begin to string into sentences.

Language is the raw material of story. Like DNA, the words we assign to experiences and the order we place them in dictate how we perceive and navigate the world. I think of all the words in this book. Trauma. Bipolar. PTSD. Madness. I think of fear and hope, love and hate, forgiveness and revenge. Depression, pain, sickness, and heartbreak. Wellness. Stasis. Happy and sad. Abuse, addiction, validation, victim, courage, and cowardice. Power and powerlessness. Agency. Surrender. Shame, success and failure, peace and war. Life itself begs for language and duality because of the comfort it provides. And because our minds love binaries, we assume that there are two stories to tell: one positive, one negative. One as victim, the other as the owner of experience. Right and wrong. Good and bad. Strong and weak. Us and them.

It's important to believe that some things are truly right and truly wrong. Believing in things anchors us. Values design our virtues and orient our moral compass. Conviction plays an essential role in purpose and purpose fulfills us. And still, what was right yesterday is often wrong now. And what is certain today will likely be questioned tomorrow. Living in the middle asks that we give our stories space to evolve, to expand, and include. We commit not to ambiguity but rather to the complexity of the human experience.

It seems silly that it needs to be said, but of course racism, sexism, xenophobia, and bigotry should be rejected. It's how people arrived at those beliefs that's worthy of curiosity. Looking there has the profound ability to validate individuals without affirming disparate beliefs. There we are interested not in a person's "truth" but the stories that led them to it. There we're all human.

A profound shift is offered if we exchange the words "but/or" with "and." It can be a biting journey that challenges a lifetime of tightly held beliefs that have defined us. But if we're brave, gentleness and forgiveness and acceptance emerge when we reject certainty for curiosity. The middle is where true love and true compassion are—and, as far as I can tell, where life is lived. The middle leads us to the truest story of everyone: *I am.* There is no duality there.

It's 2 P.M. now and I remember I haven't been outside all day. The yellow backpack I wore on Everest is right where I left it, already stuffed with a blanket and a towel. I tap my pockets for my keys and wallet and throw the pack over my shoulder.

I follow a steep staircase leading down the muddy embankment overhanging the Pacific Coast Highway. The steps are worn and bent with nails protruding from the edges and I make sure not to catch my bare feet. A broad bridge spans the noisy road and I think that everyone driving under me has their own story and they are all unique, ordinary, and extraordinary. The paths are divergent but the brain is the same: a lump of gray matter pulsing with electricity. We are all the center of our own universe. How can we not be?

The asphalt is warm under my feet as I cross the parking lot and weave through cars that are parked too close. A mother bends over a child, washing sand from his toes while he holds her shoulder for balance and asks if he might be able to have some ice cream for dinner.

I follow a wooden walkway across the broad beach until the slats disappear into the sand. The air is all tension from the promise of rain and I have no shadow as my feet blend with the earth.

I have no idea where I'm going next, but I do know I'll choose my story wisely. I'm not a climber or a photographer or a writer or a filmmaker. I want to make films. Maybe I'll write another book. Maybe I'll take a few more pictures and even climb a mountain or two. I know that I want to keep telling stories.

But now I'm thinking of my family and I hope they won't murder me for my words. I hear Mom say, "Oh, sweetheart, it is what it is," and I think I finally understand.

Somewhere my brother says, "I love you," and I let it hang in the air. Over my life I've had many brothers and sisters, but he runs through my veins and I love him fiercely. I also understand that time might not heal all wounds.

I hear Dad recite another of his favorite verses floating in his brain of limericks and songs and poems. This time it is Omar Khayyam:

The moving finger writes, and having writ moves on.
Not all the piety nor wit
Shall lure back to cancel half a line
Nor all thy tears wash out a word of it.

We can never abandon story altogether. The point is to *be mindful of the story we choose.*

I hear Dad say, "Go gently," and think it's probably time to walk home. I take another look at the Pacific. It's one of those strange, painted days when all the edges are soft and colors seem to bleed into each other. The horizon is gone and I wonder if there is really an end or beginning to anything at all. The sea and sky appear as one, losing themselves in the reflection of each other, and all the imagined black and white of the world has blended into a beautiful, seamless wash of gray. It's the color of everything.

Books end. Stories don't. Instead, they change and they change us in the process. It's strange that so much of what I've written seems like it's about someone else. The story I've told served a purpose, but the grasp of my history seems to have lost its strength. Maybe I've just learned to take my own advice. My story has changed. Hopefully, enduring stories are the ones we tell as reminders to arrive back at a few fundamentals: Be kind. Strive for presence. Change is inevitable. Listen. Stay curious. Respect nature. Above all, embrace compassion and love with abandon. It's pretty generic wisdom and I admit I sound a bit like a fortune cookie. It also seems that we all need to be reminded from time to time . . . I know I do.

I think the best stories are the ones where we exit through the same door we entered, different but the same, and I walk into my apartment and look at my life. The watch I wore in Australia sits in a shadow box on top of the small chest. The hands stopped moving almost twenty years ago. Now it reminds me of where I've been and my dual obsessions with story and time. A neat braid of purple rope that tied me to Simone and Denis on Gasherbrum II rests next to it. It's the cord that kept me tethered to this life. It bound me and unraveled me and I wonder if it was always there, hidden in plain sight. I was tied to it when I took the most impactful photograph I've ever made: a portrait of me which is a portrait of my family which is a portrait of life cascading over itself as tiny pieces of an explosion that happened 13.8 billion years ago. I look for resolution for all the loose ends and just as quickly understand that no such thing exists. Resolution is the work of words and the mind. Acceptance is the work of silence and the heart, and the space where all healing takes place. Nothing was ever broken to begin with. Broken was just another story. I am. We all are. Unbreakable.

ACKNOWLEDGMENTS

This list would be another book of pages filled only with names. It would be a pretty boring read. There are people who have influenced me more than others and I'm confident you know who you are. It might seem lazy, but a list makes no sense. I honestly believe everyone who I've encountered matters, and you are all worthy of gratitude for whatever role you played, no matter how small, painful, or marvelous it might have been. For all that is *me,* thank *you.*

ABOUT THE AUTHOR

Cory Richards is an internationally renowned photographer, filmmaker/director, and writer. In 2011, Richards became the first and only American to climb one of the world's 8,000-meter peaks in winter. His documentation of the climb and aftermath of the experience was made into the award-winning documentary *Cold* and appeared on the cover of the 125th-anniversary issue of *National Geographic*. In 2012, Richards received the prestigious designation of *National Geographic* Adventurer of the Year and in 2014 was named a *National Geographic* Photography Fellow. He is a two-time recipient of an Explorers Grant and has photographed twelve feature assignments for the magazine. Richards has an active speaking career, in which he speaks about conservation, mental health, leadership, and vulnerability.

ABOUT THE TYPE

This book was set in Caslon, a typeface first designed in 1722 by William Caslon (1692–1766). Its widespread use by most English printers in the early eighteenth century soon supplanted the Dutch typefaces that had formerly prevailed. The roman is considered a "workhorse" typeface due to its pleasant, open appearance, while the italic is exceedingly decorative.